The Immunity Plan

With over 25 years' experience in the world of nutrition, an MSc in personalized nutrition and soon a PhD, Kate Llewellyn-Waters is committed to bringing the science of nutrition and its impact on health to readers so they can achieve optimal well-being for life. She is the author of *The Immunity Cookbook* and is a presenter on *BBC Morning Live* and Channel 5's *You Are What You Eat*. Kate has had several peer-reviewed academic papers published in leading academic journals and is a reviewer for the *Journal of Qualitative Research in Sports Studies*.

Outside of work, Kate enjoys raising awareness of hearing loss, having lost 75 per cent of her hearing several years ago when pregnant with her daughter, Beatrix. With severe hearing loss and as a hearing aid wearer, Kate is committed to reducing the stigma surrounding hearing loss and the wearing of hearing aids.

The Immunity Plan

KATE LLEWELLYN-WATERS

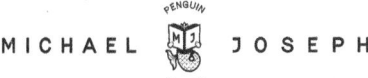

PENGUIN MICHAEL JOSEPH

UK | USA | Canada | Ireland | Australia
India | New Zealand | South Africa

Penguin Michael Joseph is part of the Penguin Random House group of companies whose addresses can be found at global.penguinrandomhouse.com

Penguin Random House UK,
One Embassy Gardens, 8 Viaduct Gardens, London SW11 7BW

penguin.co.uk

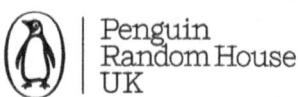

First published 2026
001

Copyright © Kate Llewellyn-Waters, 2026

The moral right of the author has been asserted

The information in this book is intended for general guidance only. While every effort has been made to ensure that the information is complete and accurate, it is not a substitute for medical or healthcare professional advice. Please consult with your GP or a qualified health professional before changing, stopping or starting any treatment or medication. All matters regarding your health require medical supervision. The author and publishers disclaim, as far as the law allows, any liability arising directly or indirectly from the use, or misuse, of the information in this book

No part of this book may be used or reproduced in any manner for the purpose of training artificial intelligence technologies or systems. In accordance with Article 4(3) of the DSM Directive 2019/790, Penguin Random House expressly reserves this work from the text and data mining exception

Set in 10.9/16pt Milo Serif Pro Text
Typeset by Six Red Marbles UK, Thetford, Norfolk
Printed and bound in Great Britain by Clays Ltd, Elcograf S.p.A.

The authorized representative in the EEA is Penguin Random House Ireland, Morrison Chambers, 32 Nassau Street, Dublin D02 YH68

A CIP catalogue record for this book is available from the British Library

ISBN: 978-0-241-79529-3

Penguin Random House is committed to a sustainable future for our business, our readers and our planet. This book is made from Forest Stewardship Council® certified paper.

Contents

Introduction   1

PART 1
The Science   9

   1 Immune System Basics   11
   2 The Autoimmunity Crisis   24
   3 Allergies and Infections   47
   4 Immunometabolism   66
   5 The Importance of the Microbiomes   76

PART 2
Evidence-Based Strategies For Improved Immunity   91

   6 The Good Gut Health Plan   93
   7 How to Eat for a Balanced Immune System – Macronutrients   106
   8 How to Eat for a Balanced Immune System – Micronutrients   131
   9 Love Your Liver   161
  10 Sort Your MESS Out!   181
  11 Should I Supplement?   213
  12 The Immunity Plan – Putting It All Together   232

PART 3
The Recipes   237

    Breakfast   239
    Lunch   249
    Dinner   269
    Sweet Treats   290

Acknowledgements   301
References   303
Index   331

For anyone who has struggled with their own invisible battles, may this book offer hope.

Introduction

We may just think of our immune system as something that only 'kicks in' during the winter months when we pick up a cold or cough; however, it actually plays a key role in lots of different aspects of our health. In fact, increasing research has shown that our immune system plays an essential role in almost **all** areas of our physical, mental and emotional health. This incredible system influences how our brain functions; impacts heart health, metabolism, gut health, inflammation levels and mood; and is continually on the 'lookout' for cancer cells.

It is clear that as we age, supporting our immune system is more important than ever. An imbalanced immune system has a significant impact on our quality of life, and can lead to chronic pain, disability, poorer mental health and, sadly, death.

Immune system disorders are on the rise, and one area of immune function that has spiralled out of control is autoimmune disease, which is the result of the immune system attacking its own tissues. There are currently over a hundred autoimmune diseases, and while the exact causes are still unknown, they are believed to involve a combination of genetics, environmental factors and poor gut health. Autoimmune disease can affect our bodies on every level with some conditions affecting the heart, endocrine glands (pancreas, adrenals and thyroid), skin, joints, muscles and even the nervous system.

> More women are affected by autoimmune disease than by breast cancer and heart disease combined.

Research indicates that women tend to have a stronger immune response than men, which, while beneficial in fighting infections more efficiently, may increase the risk of immune disorders.[1] Almost 50 per cent of women who develop an autoimmune disease do so in the first year following pregnancy; then, as a woman enters perimenopause, the decrease in female sex hormones leads to a significant decrease in immune function, resulting in a reduction to a similar level of male immune function, or even less. In addition, during perimenopause a woman's oestrogen levels decline, which switches on inflammation that can impact the gut and the immune system, thereby increasing the risk of autoimmune disease.

Women constitute approximately 78 per cent of those affected by autoimmune diseases, and around 85 per cent of people affected with **multiple** autoimmune diseases are female.[2] My own mother is one of these statistics, having been diagnosed with Sjögren's syndrome, an autoimmune disease affecting mostly women and most commonly first diagnosed in the 40s and 50s age group. This condition affects the body's exocrine glands (the glands that produce tears and saliva), with dry eyes and mouth, joint and muscle pain, and fatigue as the primary features of the condition.

I know, as my mother has Sjögren's, that I am at a greater risk of developing this disease, but for the last 25 years, armed with the nutrition and lifestyle knowledge that I am fortunate to have, I have followed the same recommendations that are included here in *The Immunity Plan*. Ensuring I have strong, balanced immunity reduces my risk of developing an autoimmune disease, such as Sjögren's syndrome.

INTRODUCTION

As an MSc-qualified nutritionist and academic researcher, I have helped hundreds of individuals improve their immune function to achieve a balanced and healthy immune system. Environmental toxins, poor diet, allergens, chronic stress, unresolved infections and imbalanced gut bacteria are believed to be the root causes of almost all immune disorders. By eliminating these aggressors, and improving immune function through nutrition, diet and lifestyle changes, research shows that you can significantly improve your immune health.

The Immunity Plan is a reference guide that will provide you with clear, easy-to-understand, scientifically proven and evidence-based diet, nutrition and lifestyle recommendations, complete with immunity-supporting recipes.

A strong, balanced and healthy immune system is our goal.

How To Use This Book

My aim is to give you the tools to understand what you can do to help support your immunity, reduce inflammation, decrease oxidative stress and minimize your risk of acquiring an immune disorder, such as autoimmune disease. However, if you are already suffering from an imbalanced immune system or a debilitating autoimmune disease, by improving your diet, nutrition and lifestyle you can, in turn, improve your immune health and potentially even reverse your symptoms.

Part 1 looks at how our immune system works and the role of the microbiome in immunity, as well as what autoimmune disease is and why women are more at risk than men.

Part 2 explores evidence-based strategies to support improved immune and gut health. We have the tools right at our fingertips to take control of our immunity and gut health, and I will guide you through the nutrition interventions that have been shown to be beneficial and address whether nutritional supplementation may be useful for you. We will explore how to optimize areas such as liver health, sleep, stress management, sunlight exposure and physical activity, as well as mental and emotional health. Also included is an easy-to-follow reference table you can refer to that summarizes all the advice in *The Immunity Plan*.

Part 3 includes immune-supporting and gut-nourishing recipes that are accessible, straightforward and inexpensive, and which the whole family can enjoy. Each recipe provides information on the different nutrients in the dish and how they benefit and support immune function and gut health. Gluten-free, dairy-free and plant-based options are included where possible.

This is an accessible guide to support you in implementing the diet and lifestyle tweaks to improve your immune and gut health for the long term.

How Healthy Is Your Immune System?

This questionnaire considers different factors that will provide you with an idea of how healthy and balanced your immune system is.

Answer the following questions and then add together the point values of each of your responses.

1. **Over the last 12 months, how would you rate your health?**
   - Very poor = 3
   - Not great = 2
   - OK = 1
   - Excellent = 0

INTRODUCTION

2. **Have you been to your doctor over the last 12 months for any health concerns?**
   - Four or more times = 3
   - Three times = 2
   - One or two times = 1
   - No times = 0

3. **Over the last 12 months, how many mild infections – such as a cold or cough – have you experienced?**
   - Seven or more = 3
   - Five or six = 2
   - Three or four = 1
   - Two or fewer = 0

The number of colds that children get a year is higher compared with adults, and some children can get up to eight colds a year.

4. **Do you have a diagnosed autoimmune condition?**
   - More than one = 3
   - Only one = 2
   - No, but I am showing symptoms = 1
   - None = 0

5. **Do you have hay fever, asthma or eczema?**
   - All of the above = 3
   - Two of the above = 2
   - One of the above = 1
   - None of the above = 0

6. **Do you have any known allergies?**
   - More than one = 3
   - Only one = 2
   - No, but I am showing symptoms = 1
   - None = 0

7. **How do you heal from wounds?**
   - Always heal poorly and slowly = 3
   - Sometimes heal slowly = 2
   - Mostly well = 1
   - Always heal well = 0

8. **On average, how many hours do you sleep each night?**
   - Less than six = 3
   - Six = 2
   - Seven = 1
   - Eight or more = 0

Results

9 or more
You have lots of areas that need support to improve the health of your immune system. Now is the time to implement these changes, and this book will guide you every step of the way to help you reach your immune health goals.

7 or 8
Your immune system seems to be struggling, and modifications to your diet and lifestyle are highly recommended to help you improve your immune health. This book will advise and guide you on how to implement these changes.

5 or 6

Your immune system appears to be functioning adequately but not optimally, and there is room for improvement. To support your immunity even further, check where you scored highly and focus on making changes in these areas. There are plenty of lifestyle and diet implementations that will support your immune health.

4 or less

Fantastic! It sounds like your immune system is strong, balanced, efficient and healthy. To continue to optimize your health, check where you scored highly and focus on making lifestyle improvements in these areas.

Let's begin!

PART 1

The Science

CHAPTER 1

Immune System Basics

The immune system is highly complex and is often thought of as the body's main defence system. It is made up of numerous organs as well as different tissues, cells and cell subtypes that work, in synergy, as a team. Your clever immune system is at work every minute of the day, protecting you and reacting constantly to your internal and external environment.

However, your immune system is doing much more than just defending against harmful 'invaders' such as bacteria, viruses and fungi. Studies have shown that it is involved in various bodily processes such as cancer surveillance, metabolism, brain function and mood. In fact, your immune system is involved in almost all aspects of health – physical, emotional and mental. Therefore, focusing on improving your immunity is not just for fighting off these potentially harmful pathogens in the short term but for *life*.

Let's think of the tissues, cells and molecules in our immune system as a sports team – they all have different but vital roles to play.

The Cells

White Blood Cells

White blood cells, also known as leucocytes, are the most common of our immune cells. There are several types of white blood cells, including neutrophils, monocytes, lymphocytes, basophils and eosinophils.

If any harmful bacteria, virus or other pathogen enters our body, then the white blood cells swiftly kick into action, identifying the pathogen and subsequently fighting off this potentially harmful invader.

Lymphocytes are very capable white blood cells that can destroy pathogens efficiently. Two types of lymphocytes are known as B lymphocytes and T lymphocytes and are made in our bone marrow. Some cells move from the bone marrow to the thymus (a gland behind our sternum), where they then become T cells, while other cells remain and become B cells. The role of the T cells is to regulate the immune response and help combat cancer cells, while the role of the B cells is to make antibodies (protective proteins), created by the immune system to combat an antigen (something that incites an antibody response).

> **Antibodies** are proteins produced by the immune system which protect you when an unwanted substance, such as a bacteria or virus, enters your body.
>
> **Antigens** are foreign substances which provoke an antibody response. They can include bacteria, viruses, fungi and toxins. An allergy-inducing food, such as shellfish, egg or milk, can also be an antigen.

If we do not produce an abundance of varied T and B cells – which is what occurs during ageing – our immune system may miss certain bacteria, viruses or other invaders. These can then remain and potentially lead to illness and disease.

The natural killer cells, known as NK cells, are another type of lymphocyte. They make up 10 per cent of our white blood cells and are spread out in different places in our body, such as the lymph nodes, lungs and liver. These cells are fast to fight potentially harmful pathogens and destroy virus-infected cells. Our NK cells do this by determining alterations that occur in our body's cells when a virus infects them. These powerful cells are also busy carrying out continual surveillance for the presence of cancer cells and investigate every cell carefully.

We also have our regulatory T cells (Tregs), and these are our main peacekeepers and control the other immune cells. Tregs shut down the immune reaction at the end of an immune response after the other immune cells have played their role. Tregs are vital for a balanced immune system, as an imbalanced immune system may lead to chronic inflammation, reduced energy, poorer mental health and accelerated ageing. In addition, Tregs are in charge of signalling whether our immune system should withdraw, halt the assault and step down. We need to ensure our Tregs regulate appropriately and effectively but not excessively. Too many Tregs can result in inadequate immunity, which may lead to increased infections and cancer risk, while not enough Tregs may result in excessive regulation, resulting in our cells and organs being potentially damaged.

Some of this is determined by our genetics, but fortunately, we are able to take control by making the best nutrition and lifestyle choices we can, and by ensuring adequate physical activity, sleep and effective stress management.

> Every single day, the human body manufactures and destroys approximately **100 billion** neutrophils – the most common type of white blood cell and the body's first line of defence.

Red Blood Cells

These cells are made in our bone marrow and contain a protein called haemoglobin, which carries oxygen from the lungs to all parts of the body. However, when it comes to their role in immunity, research shows red blood cells' immune functions to be diverse. They bind to potentially harmful pathogens, and in some cases they release oxygen from their haemoglobin to kill bacteria in a process called oxycytosis. This is a quick and effective process that kills bacteria and removes them from the bloodstream.

The Lymphatic System

The lymphatic system is an important part of our immune system and involves tissues and organs that help the body fight infection and disease. The lymphatic system runs through the entire body, carrying a fluid known as lymph, and helps our body eliminate toxins and waste. Our diligent white blood cells also use lymph to carry out their important surveillance, so they are ready to destroy any foreign substances that may cause us potential harm.

Lymphatic Vessels and Lymph Nodes

This intricate system consists of tube-like lymphatic vessels and lymph nodes (bean-shaped organs) which filter the lymph. We have approximately 500–600 lymph nodes that store our immune cells, and it is here that our immune cells can explore for any potential pathogens that may be lurking.

Have you ever felt swollen lymph nodes when you have been ill? You may have felt them at the side of your neck if you have had a throat infection or cold. They swell as a response to an infection due to the presence of immune cells, bacteria and lymph. In addition to the sides of the neck, you may feel them enlarged under your armpits or in the groin area.

Unlike our blood, which is pumped around the body, the lymphatic fluid is squeezed though the vessels when our muscles are activated, so physical activity is essential to allow lymph to move and for immune health. Our lymph vessels have valves that ensure that the lymph is moving, and the valves are one-way, which prevents any lymph moving backwards.

Bone Marrow

Bone marrow is the tissue in our bones that contains stem cells and is essential for producing blood cells that are involved in immune function. Most immune cells after early childhood are produced in the bone marrow.

Spleen

The spleen is an organ located in the upper-left abdomen and its role is to regulate the level of blood cells, remove old and damaged blood cells, and destroy harmful germs. Sometimes, an individual may need their spleen to be removed; however, if this happens, then the liver is able to take control of the spleen's functions, and we can live without it.

Thymus

The thymus gland is situated behind the breastbone (sternum), and despite being active only until puberty, it has a vital role when it is active and supports the body in preventing autoimmunity (when the immune system mounts an attack against its own cells and tissues). During childhood, the thymus is involved in producing our T lymphocytes, which are crucial for immune health. Our thymus is at its largest in childhood, and after puberty it begins to get smaller; by the age of 75, it is basically little more than fatty tissue.

Tonsils

Tonsils are lymphoid tissue located near the entrance of the digestive and respiratory tracts at the back of the throat, and they play an essential role in our immune system. There are two tonsils, one on each side, and are the front line of defence that form the initial immune response to an inhaled or ingested pathogen.

Adenoids

Along with the tonsils, adenoids form an important part of the lymphatic system. Adenoids are small masses of lymphoid tissue that are situated at the back of the nasal passage, also known as the nasopharynx. Adenoids are an important part of the immune system, helping to fight infection by trapping the harmful germs that enter through the mouth and nose. They typically begin to shrink when we're around four years old and disappear by early adulthood.

The Innate And Adaptive Immune Systems

Our immune system is like a very sophisticated security set-up that consists of two different teams. The first team is our innate immunity, which acts as the rapid-response team and provides immediate defence by launching a powerful response against potentially harmful pathogens. The second team is our adaptive immunity, the highly trained and specialized team that, from its previous experiences, has developed to protect us even more competently and effectively in the future. These two teams must work together to maintain health; when the balance is threatened, we are at an increased risk of infections as well as chronic inflammation and autoimmune disease.

> **Immune modulation** is the process of refining the immune response so that our whole immune system works together in harmony.

The innate immune system is our immediate first line of defence – the initial stage in an immune response – and involves a varied assortment of white blood cells and molecules. Innate immunity is activated when we fall and hurt ourselves, inflammation and tissue damage occur and we feel pain; however, it is also involved in removing cells that are malfunctioning or old.

> Our immune system has two arms – the **innate** and **adaptive** – working on their own and together to maintain our health.

When our innate immune system cannot sort the issue out, our second line of defence – which is known as adaptive immunity – is activated. This arm of our immune system can take some time to kick into action – around five days to a week – and is controlled by our lymphocytes, namely the B and T lymphocytes. Our innate immune cells, called phagocytes, present antigens that the adaptive immune system can recognize; it then assembles the T cells to launch an immune response.

We can look at the innate immune system like an alarm clock going off: it awakens the adaptive immune system. During adaptive immunity, our immune cells are acting as surveillants and keeping an eye out in case we are infected with a germ we have previously encountered that needs destroying. This frequently occurs without us knowing and even before we have presented with any signs of illness.

Our genes are an essential consideration here, as our human leucocyte antigen (HLA) immunity genes differ massively between us, which illustrates how we are all highly unique when it comes to our immune systems. Understanding HLA genes is complicated, but it is vital I explain this briefly as it is the reason why we all react in different ways to the same infection. Take the virus SARS-CoV-2, for example, which caused the disease Covid-19. A close friend and I responded very differently to that same virus – why did this happen? Well, our immune systems may launch an efficient response to the virus, but how competently our T and B cells execute this will be determined to some extent by our individual HLA molecules as these influence how efficiently we can turn on our adaptive immune response.[1]

Our adaptive immune system is incredibly clever; it is like a memory bank, remembering and 'archiving' all the past viral and bacterial infections we have encountered, and is able to recognize them by their molecular shape. This is what we refer to as immunological memory and it is like an elephant – it does not tend to forget!

Immunological Memory

This is one of the most important elements of the immune response – its ability to recall previous infections is vital since the immune system will then be able to respond more effectively and rapidly to germs that you have previously encountered. Your immunological memory is the reason you catch certain diseases like chickenpox once, even though you may have been exposed to it numerous times. Unfortunately, there are some devious culprits like rhinovirus, which is the cause of the common cold, that have established clever tactics to bypass our immunological memory. They do this by constantly altering their molecular information and recognition code on their surfaces.

Fortunately, immunological memory can last a very long time, and a 2016 study demonstrated that for the research participants who were analysed, their memory of the measles infection would take more than 3,000 years to decrease by half.[2] These lasting changes are the reason why vaccines offer predominantly long-lasting protection. However, vaccines do vary, so the exact type of memory produced by different vaccines may differ significantly. Furthermore, individuals respond differently to vaccines, as we saw with the Covid-19 vaccine, due to variations in genes, age and environmental factors.

As with everything immune-system related, we need **balance**, and issues may arise if the adaptive immune response is inappropriately triggered, which as we will discover in the next chapter can lead to significant adverse effects.

As I mentioned earlier in this chapter, our immune system impacts many different areas of our health – let's take a closer look at these.

Brain Health

Our immune system plays a vital role in supporting a healthy brain, where special immune cells called microglia are the first line of defence. These cells help eliminate potentially harmful substances and are continually looking out for any damage or disease. However, when the immune system 'malfunctions' this can contribute to the development of neurodegenerative issues or dementia. In conditions such as Alzheimer's and other types of dementia, the immune response becomes chronically activated, which can lead to significant issues.

In addition, research has shown that numerous genes that are associated with a greater risk of dementia are active in the immune cells of the brain, thereby indicating their significance in Alzheimer's and other forms of dementia.

Inflammation

Inflammation anywhere in the body can also affect brain health, and systemic inflammation present in conditions such as obesity, cardiovascular disease and type 2 diabetes can impact the blood–brain barrier and also increase the risk of neurodegenerative issues. The blood–brain barrier plays a vital role in protecting the brain, so we need to ensure we minimize inflammation as much as possible. Fortunately, this can be achieved with the appropriate nutrition and lifestyle choices – all of which is in our control.

Metabolism

In short, metabolism is a process that converts what we eat and drink into energy, and metabolic processes can impact how our immune cells function. We have known for a long time from the available research that any 'disturbances' to metabolism, including obesity, are also associated with immune system changes such as inflammation.[3] The term 'immunometabolism' was coined in 2011 in a *Nature* journal article [4] to explain the complex relationship between the immune system and metabolism, and we will look at the importance of immunometabolism in Chapter 4.

It is very clear that our immune system and metabolic system are closely connected. Our metabolism supports the high energy requirements of our immune cells, and at the same time, our immune system and any inflammatory immune responses can significantly influence metabolic homeostasis. This can potentially increase our risk of several health conditions, such as obesity and type 2 diabetes, if not functioning appropriately.

> **Metabolic homeostasis** means reaching and maintaining a state of metabolic balance.

Heart Health

The heart and the immune system are also very closely connected, with the immune system supporting heart health by helping to repair tissue damage as well as promoting the formation of new blood vessels and removing harmful pathogens.

Immune cells are essential after a cardiac injury for the initial wound healing response; however, excessive immune responses can worsen any heart damage and contribute to conditions such as atherosclerosis. This is a condition where fatty plaques build up in arteries, and if left unmanaged, it can ultimately lead to an increased risk of stroke or heart attacks.

Acute inflammation is the body's immediate response to

infection or injury where there are symptoms such as swelling, heat, pain or redness. It is a protective process that will help remove damaged tissue or bring immune cells to combat the harmful invader/irritant and allow the healing process to start. Chronic inflammation, meanwhile, is a long-term state of inflammation which can damage our body's healthy tissue and lead to diseases such as type 2 diabetes, heart disease, cancer and autoimmune disease. Ensuring chronic inflammation is kept to a minimum is essential, and this can be achieved by making the best nutrition and lifestyle choices possible.

Gut Health

Our gut microbiome and our immune system are intricately linked, with the microbiome shaping immune cell development and function, and in turn, the immune system helps to maintain optimal gut health. The gut is actually the largest immunological organ, housing the majority of the body's immune cells. As we will explore in more detail in Chapter 5, a balanced microbiome helps to promote a healthy immune system that is capable of maintaining tolerance to the body's own tissues, limiting the risk of autoimmune disease as well as effectively eliminating any potentially harmful pathogens.

Summary

Our immune system, as we have seen, is made up of lots of different cells, tissues and organs. It has many roles, including protecting us against potentially harmful bacteria, viruses and fungi; surveilling for cancer cells; supporting our metabolism, brain function, heart health and gut health; and regulating inflammation levels.

This incredible system is involved in almost all areas of health, and improving our immune health will not just help to fight off harmful pathogens in the short term but will also help support almost every other system in our body for life. If we look after our immunity, it will look after us!

CHAPTER 2

The Autoimmunity Crisis

On a daily basis, we are faced with numerous potentially very harmful pathogens. Our immune systems are dealing with these threats quietly and efficiently without us realizing as we go on with the rest of our day.

Autoimmune Disease

It is not only potential infections that our immune systems are having to deal with continually: our own immune systems may cause us harm due to the risk of autoimmune disease, which is currently at epidemic levels.

Autoimmunity is when our immune system begins to attack our healthy cells, which then leads to a loss of tolerance to the self, and when our own tissues and organs are attacked and damaged. Unfortunately, the result of this happening is autoimmune disease. At present, researchers believe there are between 80 and 150 autoimmune diseases.[1]

> **Autoimmune conditions** are the result of the immune system attacking its own tissues, which leads to increased inflammation and oxidative stress as well as accelerated immunological ageing.

Autoimmune disease may affect different parts of the body. While some autoimmune disorders are organ-specific – such as in type 1 diabetes, which impacts the pancreas – other autoimmune diseases can cause harm to other areas of the body, such as lupus, which may affect the heart, lungs, joints and skin. This can result in long-term pain, fatigue, low energy and poor mental health.

A study published in the *Lancet* medical journal involving 22 million people in the UK reported that autoimmune disorders now affect approximately one in ten individuals. Among the 22 million individuals included in the study, 978,872 had a new diagnosis of at least one autoimmune disease between 2000 and 2019.[2] In the United States, it is a similar situation: it is believed that 8 per cent of the population are living with an autoimmune disease, and approximately 80 per cent of these diseases are diagnosed in women.[3] Worryingly, autoimmune disease prevalence is increasing and the cost to manage these disorders is costing the economy billions annually.

> **Autoimmune diseases** are identified by the chronic inflammation and tissue damage resulting from unregulated immune responses throughout the body.

Why Do Autoimmune Diseases Happen?

An autoimmune disease is not caused by one single factor but by numerous factors. This has been defined as the 'mosaic of autoimmunity', which is an interaction between our genes and other factors, with many still unknown.[4] And while the precise reason as to why acquiring an autoimmune disease occurs is not fully known, it is thought to be due to genetics, environmental factors, a poor gut microbiome and compromised gut-barrier health.

> **The mosaic of autoimmunity** refers to the different combinations of many factors involved in autoimmunity that result in different symptoms and signs, representing the wide spectrum of autoimmune diseases.[5]

Research has indicated that genetic predisposition may explain approximately 30 per cent of all autoimmune conditions while a whopping 70 per cent are due to environmental aggressors, such as exposure to toxins and chemicals, poor diet, infections, chronic stress and gut dysbiosis (an imbalance in the gut bacteria).[6]

It is important to get a suspected autoimmune disease diagnosed as early as possible, as left unmanaged it could lead to an erratic and non-functional immune system. This could then increase the risk of acquiring a further autoimmune disease, which is known as polyautoimmunity. Unfortunately, some individuals have three or more autoimmune disorders, which is known as multiple autoimmune syndrome (MAS).

Autoimmune disease is still a fairly poorly understood area, but these debilitating and life-changing disorders can affect our bodies on every level, impacting the heart, pancreas, thyroid, skin, joints, muscles and even the nervous system. Autoimmune diseases are also associated with other health conditions, such as heart disease, cancer and sleep apnoea. Sadly, many people suffer in silence for several years, with the autoimmune disease continuing to cause significant damage to the individual. In fact, it is believed that a diagnosis can take approximately four and a half years.

> **Autoimmune disease** is one of the main causes of mortality in those under 75 years old in the UK.

As I touched on in the introduction, we also know that hormonal fluctuations can significantly impact the likelihood of developing an autoimmune disease.

Common Autoimmune Diseases

Some of the most common autoimmune diseases include rheumatoid arthritis, lupus, coeliac disease, multiple sclerosis, Hashimoto's disease, type 1 diabetes and Sjögren's syndrome.

RHEUMATOID ARTHRITIS

In rheumatoid arthritis (RA) the immune system sends antibodies to the lining of the joints by accident and then these antibodies attack the tissues surrounding the joints. This causes the thin layer of cells (synovium) covering the joints to become inflamed, which is painful. In addition, inflammation causes chemicals to be released which thicken the synovium and may cause damage to the bones, cartilage (connective tissue between bones that protects them), tendons (connects bone to muscle) and ligaments (connects bone to bone). These chemicals may also alter the shape of the joint over time. RA is the most common inflammatory arthritis, and the confirmed prevalence of the disease is approximately 1 per cent of the UK population, which is similar to worldwide prevalence. Like many autoimmune conditions, RA is two to four times more common in women than in men, and onset of the disease can occur at any age but tends to start between the ages of 30 and 50. RA that starts after the age of 60 is called late-onset rheumatoid arthritis (LORA).

> Family history of rheumatoid arthritis confers a **two- to four-fold increase** in risk for first-degree relatives.[7]

There are many symptoms an individual with RA may present with, such as:

- pain
- swelling
- heat around the joints
- redness
- stiffness and difficulty moving the affected joints
- nodules over a swollen joint and under the skin
- tiredness
- high temperature
- low-grade fever
- low mood
- sweating
- poor appetite
- weight loss.

Blood tests may determine if you have RA, and one blood test that measures the inflammatory marker, C-reactive protein (CRP), will confirm how much inflammation is present at that current time.

Living with RA can be hard as often the symptoms are unpredictable. There is no way of knowing when a flare-up will happen, with the stiffness and pain being worse some days than others. This unpredictability can lead to increased anxiety and stress levels and potentially low mood and poorer mental health. Approximately one third of people have to stop working because of the condition within two years of onset of the disease. Fortunately, certain treatments can help ease symptoms, such as physiotherapy, which can help to increase muscle strength, flexibility and fitness. Occupational therapy can also be of benefit as it provides training and advice if you need help with everyday tasks or are having difficulty at work.

The risk of acquiring RA increases with age, so looking after our immune system as we age is vital.

LUPUS

Also known as systemic lupus erythematosus, this disorder involves multiple bodily tissues due to the body making antibodies against our DNA, a fundamental component of cells. This then leads to inflammation and potential damage in various tissues and organs.

Research shows that around 90 per cent of lupus sufferers tend to be female, and it is most common in women of childbearing age – approximately 16 to 50 years old. The causes of lupus are not fully understood, but possible causes include a viral infection, sunlight, puberty, childbirth and menopause. The hormone oestrogen is also thought to play a significant role, while some medications can also cause lupus-like side effects.

> **Lupus** tends to be less common in people of white European origin and more common in people of African, Caribbean or Asian origin.[8]

Symptoms of lupus are wide-ranging and may include:

- muscle pain
- extreme tiredness that won't go away
- mouth ulcers
- rashes that usually come on after being in the sun – the rash is often over the nose and cheeks
- high temperature or fever (during a flare-up)
- hair loss
- weight loss
- swollen glands, usually in the neck, armpits or groin
- low mood and anxiety

- chest pain
- stomach pain
- changes in the colour of your fingers and toes when you are cold, anxious or stressed.[9]

If lupus is suspected, then your medical practitioner will carry out some blood tests, one of which is the antinuclear antibodies (ANA) test. However, a positive test does not necessarily mean you have lupus as other tests also need to be conducted. These investigations include testing for antiphospholipid antibodies, antibodies to double-stranded DNA and anti-Smith antibodies. A rheumatologist will consider the test results as well as signs, symptoms and medical history to confirm a diagnosis. Sometimes someone with lupus may be referred for an X-ray and scan, which is conducted to assess whether the heart, kidneys or any other organs may be affected.

COELIAC DISEASE

As a nutritionist, I see a lot of individuals who have coeliac disease. In this condition, the villi, which are like tiny fingers lining the inside of your small intestine, become damaged. This can happen over many years of eating foods containing gluten before a coeliac disease diagnosis is made. Gluten may also impact other organs, so an individual can experience many different symptoms, such as tiredness, low thyroid function, brain fog, anaemia and arthritis.

An antibodies blood test will be carried out to check for coeliac disease. It is important to continue to include gluten in your diet when the blood test is done because avoiding it could lead to an inaccurate result. If coeliac disease antibodies are found in your blood, then you may require more blood tests, or a biopsy of your intestine may be performed. However, it is not uncommon for an individual to have coeliac disease and not have these antibodies in their blood.

Sometimes additional blood tests may be required to see how the condition has affected you, such as measuring the levels of iron to check whether coeliac disease has caused other issues, including iron deficiency anaemia (a lack of iron in the blood) from nutrients being poorly absorbed. Some individuals may present with dermatitis herpetiformis, which is an itchy rash, and in these cases a skin biopsy may be carried out under local anaesthetic, involving a small skin sample being taken so it can be examined under a microscope. Bone health may also be affected, due to the poor absorption of nutrients, which may make bones weaker and more brittle. If a medical practitioner suspects this, then a DEXA scan (a type of X-ray) may be advised; this will measure bone density to see if you are at an increased risk of bone fractures.

MULTIPLE SCLEROSIS

Our body's nerves are covered by a protective coating called myelin, and in MS sufferers, the myelin in the brain and spinal cord is damaged. The most frequently seen initial symptom is dysfunction of the central nervous system, and a condition that causes pain in the eye (optic neuritis) can be a first symptom of MS. In optic neuritis, the pain can worsen as you move the eye in different directions, and other eye issues such as blurred vision may also occur. Symptoms may flare up and then go into remission and, frequently, symptoms may get worse over time.

Other symptoms include:

- a tingling, pins-and-needles or numbness feeling in different parts of the body
- feeling dizzy or uncoordinated and clumsy
- swelling
- muscle cramps, spasms or stiffness

- itching
- fatigue
- needing to urinate more frequently
- cognitive, memory or concentration issues
- sexual problems, such as vaginal dryness or erectile dysfunction.

If your medical practitioner suspects you may have MS, they will refer you to a brain and nerve specialist, known as a neurologist. While there is no single, definitive test to diagnose MS, an MRI scan which looks for lesions or damage to the nerves in the brain or spinal cord may be conducted. A lumbar puncture may also be carried out, which involves taking a small sample of spinal fluid from your lower back using a needle.

Tests to measure coordination, movement, balance, reflexes and vision will be conducted. Other screening includes blood tests and potentially tests that use small sensors that are attached to your skin to assess how quickly messages from your ears or eyes travel to your brain.

> Multiple sclerosis risk factors:
> - you are 20–50 years old
> - you are female
> - you have a sister, brother or parent with MS
> - you smoke (people who smoke are about twice as likely to develop the disease)
> - you have had the Epstein–Barr virus, which causes glandular fever, in the past.

THE AUTOIMMUNITY CRISIS

While there is presently no cure for MS, there are treatments that can slow the progression of the condition and help to ease symptoms. Physiotherapy can help with movement issues and muscular pain, and cognitive behavioural therapy (CBT) may help with low mood, anxiety and tiredness. Your doctor or medical practitioner can also advise on treatments for sexual issues such as vaginal dryness or erectile dysfunction.

HASHIMOTO'S DISEASE

Hashimoto's disease was first described by a Japanese doctor in 1912 and is a common cause of hypothyroidism (an underactive thyroid). Also known as chronic autoimmune thyroiditis, Hashimoto's disease is a common autoimmune disorder that occurs when the immune system makes antibodies that attack the thyroid gland. In short, the thyroid gets infiltrated by large numbers of white blood cells and slowly becomes damaged, losing its function and ability to make a sufficient amount of thyroid hormones. These hormones are vital as they control how your body uses energy, so they impact almost every organ in your body, including the way your heart beats. In Hashimoto's, an individual will often present with an enlarged thyroid (goitre), and when the thyroid is inflamed a sore throat may also be present. A goitre may create a feeling of fullness in your throat, although it is usually not painful. After many years, damage to the thyroid may cause the gland to shrink and the goitre to disappear.

Other symptoms of Hashimoto's disease include:

- weight gain
- tiredness
- potential hair loss
- issues tolerating the cold

- joint and muscle pain
- dry skin or dry, thinning hair
- heavy or irregular menstrual periods
- fertility problems
- slowed heart rate
- constipation.

Researchers do not fully know why some individuals develop Hashimoto's disease, but a family history of thyroid disease is common. Other factors that may also play a role include genetic predisposition and exposure to viruses such as hepatitis C; it may also be triggered by stress as well as pregnancy.[10] It is four to ten times more common in women than men, and while Hashimoto's can occur at any age, it most often develops in women aged 30 to 50.[11]

Tests to investigate suspected Hashimoto's measure thyroid hormone levels, such as TSH, free T4, free T3 and anti-thyroglobulin and anti-thyroid peroxidase antibodies.

> **TSH** is produced by the pituitary gland and stimulates the thyroid to produce T3 and T4. Elevated TSH often indicates hypothyroidism (underactive thyroid), while low TSH can suggest hyperthyroidism (overactive thyroid).
>
> **Free T3** is the active form of the thyroid hormone that directly impacts the body's metabolism. Measuring free T3 helps assess thyroid hormone levels and can be used to diagnose and monitor hyperthyroidism and hypothyroidism.
>
> **Free T4** is the main thyroid hormone produced by the thyroid gland, and measuring it helps assess thyroid hormone levels and diagnose thyroid disorder.

Hashimoto's disease can be diagnosed by the presence of antibodies, increased TSH and low blood levels of thyroid hormones. You may not need other tests to confirm you have Hashimoto's disease; however, if your medical practitioner suspects the condition but you don't have anti-thyroid antibodies in your blood, you may have an ultrasound scan of your thyroid. These images will show the size of your thyroid and other features of Hashimoto's disease. The scan can also eliminate other causes of an enlarged thyroid, such as thyroid nodules, which are small lumps.

The thyroid uses iodine, a mineral in some foods, to make thyroid hormones. If you have Hashimoto's disease or other types of autoimmune thyroid disorders, you may be sensitive to harmful side effects from iodine. Eating foods that contain significant amounts of iodine, such as kelp or other kinds of seaweed, may cause hypothyroidism or worsen it. Taking iodine supplements may have the same impact; however, if you are pregnant, you need to ensure you have adequate iodine intake, as your baby gets iodine from what you consume. As with everything nutrition and health related, balance is key – too much iodine can cause problems as well, such as a goitre in the baby, so if you are pregnant or looking to become pregnant, then it is important to discuss with your medical practitioner or doctor the amount of iodine you need to consume.

In the early stages of this disease the thyroid may still be making a sufficient amount of hormones, so this is the ideal time to follow the guidance in this book to improve your immune health. You can stop the condition from worsening and actually reverse it, which will also prevent long-term damage to your thyroid.

TYPE 1 DIABETES

Type 1 diabetes causes the insulin-producing beta cells in the pancreas to become damaged, and this leads to the body being unable to produce enough insulin to adequately regulate blood glucose levels. Since type 1 diabetes results in the loss of insulin production, an individual with the condition needs to administer regular insulin, either by injection or by insulin pump. This condition used to be referred to as 'juvenile diabetes', a term which is now regarded as outdated as while the disease is frequently diagnosed in children, the condition can develop at any age. However, type 1 diabetes does tend to develop more slowly in adults than it does in children, and in some cases type 1 diabetes in adults may be misdiagnosed as type 2 diabetes; unlike type 1 diabetes, which is an autoimmune disease, type 2 diabetes is a metabolic disorder that occurs when the body can't use the insulin (a hormone that regulates blood glucose) it produces effectively, or when the pancreas doesn't produce enough insulin. Type 1 diabetes in adults over 35 years old will sometimes be referred to as latent autoimmune diabetes of adulthood (LADA).

> **Type 1 diabetes** can be affected by genetics. If your parents or siblings have type 1 diabetes, you may be at a greater risk of developing it:
>
> - **8 per cent** risk if the father has type 1 diabetes
> - **2 per cent** risk if the mother has type 1 diabetes
> - **30 per cent** risk if both parents have it.[12]

Common symptoms of type 1 diabetes include increased thirst, fatigue during the day, the need to urinate frequently, unintentional weight loss and itching in the genitals. If you have suspected diabetes, your medical practitioner may carry out blood or urine tests, such as a ketone test, GAD antibodies test and C-peptide test, to investigate whether you have the condition.

SJÖGREN'S SYNDROME

Sjögren's (pronounced Show-grin's) syndrome occurs when the immune cells attack the mucus-secreting glands, resulting in a reduction in secretions. This autoimmune disease is named after Henrik Sjögren, an ophthalmologist from Sweden, who initially identified this syndrome. Again, as in other autoimmune diseases, it is mostly women who are affected, with an estimated 90 per cent of those suffering with the condition female, and it most commonly affects people aged 40 to 60 years old. However, it is tricky to confirm exactly how many individuals have Sjögren's because many people who may have the condition do not go to see their medical practitioner about their symptoms.

In addition to the most common symptoms of dry eyes and dry mouth, other symptoms of Sjögren's include tiredness, cognitive changes, and joint and muscle pain. Dryness may also be noted in the sinuses, lungs, skin, gastrointestinal tract and vagina, as the glands that keep the vagina moist can also be affected.

Sjögren's syndrome has two forms:

- primary Sjögren's syndrome, which develops in the absence of any existing underlying condition
- secondary Sjögren's syndrome, which develops in addition to existing autoimmune diseases such as lupus, psoriatic arthritis and rheumatoid arthritis.

The reasons for Sjögren's syndrome affecting some individuals remains unknown, but research suggests that it's triggered by a combination of genetic, environmental and, potentially, hormonal factors. Also, some individuals are believed to be more at risk of acquiring Sjögren's due to certain exposures, such as an infection, which may trigger the problems with the immune system.

In the UK, tests used to diagnose Sjögren's syndrome include the tear break-up time and Schirmer tests, which are usually carried out by an ophthalmologist. The tear break-up time test measures how effective your tear glands are. A non-toxic dye is dropped on to the surface of your eye and the colour of the dye allows the ophthalmologist to see how well your tear film is functioning and how long it takes for your tears to evaporate. In the Schirmer test, small strips of blotting paper are placed into your lower eyelid. After five minutes, the strips are removed to see how much of the paper is soaked with tears.

A lip biopsy may also be conducted, which is when a small tissue sample is removed from your inner lip and examined under a microscope. A local anaesthetic is injected into the inner surface of your lower lip to numb the area before a small cut is made to remove a few of your minor salivary glands. Clusters of lymphocytes (a type of white blood cell) in the tissue can determine if you have Sjögren's syndrome.[13]

A salivary flow rate test can be carried out to measure how much saliva your glands produce. You'll usually be asked to spit as much saliva as you can into a cup over a five-minute period, and the amount of saliva is then weighed or measured. An unusually low flow rate can indicate Sjögren's syndrome. There are also blood tests that test for Sjögren's, including ANA, anti-SSA and anti-SSB antibody tests.

Currently, there is no cure for Sjögren's syndrome, but treatments can help to manage symptoms; dry eyes, for example, can be eased with artificial tears. Good eye and mouth hygiene is key because if you have Sjögren's, your risk of developing an infection is greater. Taking care of your eyes and mouth can help prevent problems such as corneal ulcers and tooth decay. At times, Sjögren's syndrome may lead to complications such as eyesight being permanently damaged if the decreased tear production isn't well managed. Also, women who have Sjögren's are at a greater risk of having children with a temporary 'lupus' rash or heart abnormalities. Therefore, if you have Sjögren's, it is important to monitor your pregnancy closely to keep an eye out for any potential issues.

Are Genes to Blame?

The majority of autoimmune diseases are polygenic, meaning that a combination of autoimmune genes may be a cause of the disease, not just one lone culprit. Although the majority of the recognized autoimmune genes are connected to the immune system somehow, we saw in the previous chapter that our immunity human leucocyte antigen (HLA) genes play an important role. How our HLA genes act means that every individual is potentially at risk of acquiring an autoimmune disease due to how our immune system has evolved. This may be a consequence of our protective immune system making immune cells which can determine a vast variety of germs' molecular codes.

While we cannot change our genes, we can control how they are 'expressed' or switched on or off.[14] This is called epigenetics and is influenced by our diet, nutrition, exercise, lifestyle and environmental choices. You may have heard the phrase, 'Your genes load the gun, but environment pulls the trigger,' and when it comes to our immunity, it is not determined totally by our genes. Instead, it is continually shaped by our changing environment and adapting to how we live.[15] Fortunately, we have control over most of our environmental factors, such as what and how we eat and drink, when and how we move, and how we manage stress and sleep. These nutrition and lifestyle decisions are up to us.

> **Epigenetics** is the study of changes in organisms caused by modification of gene expression rather than alteration of the genetic code itself.

Despite research confirming that predisposing genes do play a role in autoimmune disease, we still do not know fully how genetics are involved. However, having a family member with an autoimmune condition does increase your risk of also acquiring an autoimmune condition.

Why Are Women Affected More?

In the United States approximately 80 per cent of all autoimmune disease cases affect women, and at least 85 per cent of individuals with more than one autoimmune disease are female. Why is this? Well, research shows that in general, women tend to have a stronger immune response, which, while beneficial in beating infections more quickly, may increase the risk of immune disorders.[16]

In addition, research suggests that there are numerous genes involved in the immune response on the X chromosome, and women have two X chromosomes while men have one – women simply have more of these immune genes. However, genes alone are not enough to cause autoimmune disease, so what else is causing women to be at a greater risk of developing an autoimmune disorder?

One reason is believed to be due to sex hormones, which have been confirmed to play a key role in autoimmunity in women, and the significant endocrinological changes experienced by women at least twice during their lifetime – puberty and menopause. Many women also experience an extra hormonal transition – pregnancy, potentially accompanied by breastfeeding. These endocrinological changes have significant impacts on the immune system due to the interaction between the hormonal environment, innate and adaptive immune systems, and pro- and anti-inflammatory cytokines, which are small proteins that play an important role in immune function.

Sex hormones, such as oestrogen and progesterone, are frequently implicated in an increased risk of autoimmune disorders because of their complex interactions with the immune system. Furthermore, sex hormones can directly impact immune cells, such as T cells and B cells, as well as Tregs, which we know are vital for maintaining self-tolerance as they suppress the immune system to prevent it from attacking the body's own cells and tissues. Additionally, the female sex hormone, oestrogen, has a complicated role when it comes to inflammation as it has a pro-inflammatory effect that may increase the immune response and the risk of autoimmunity in women. On the other hand, oestrogen also has an anti-inflammatory effect and can inhibit certain cells while increasing other cells, such as Tregs, which help to suppress excessive immune responses. Meanwhile, androgens, such as testosterone, are generally considered to play a protective role against autoimmunity, and animal studies have indicated that testosterone and dihydrotestosterone can suppress immune responses and inflammation.

> Almost **50 per cent of women** who develop an autoimmune disease do so in the first 12 months following pregnancy.

As a woman enters perimenopause, the decrease in female sex hormones leads to a significant reduction in immune function, resulting in a decrease that is comparable to a similar level of male immune function or potentially even less.[17] Despite this, autoimmune diseases are very rarely discussed as a women's health issue. Thus, as we age, supporting our immune system and hormonal balance is more important than ever. Further research and a deeper understanding of hormonal changes and their potential role on immune function and autoimmune diseases is urgently needed.

This may help to potentially predict, prevent and possibly cure these debilitating diseases that are most prevalent in women.[18]

Ultimately, ensuring we keep our hormones as balanced as possible is key. When hormone levels become imbalanced, this impacts not only our immune system but also our gut microbiome and other bodily functions that are involved in the development of autoimmune disease. Fortunately, we can achieve healthy hormonal balance by consuming a nutritious and diverse diet, reducing added sugar intake, maintaining a healthy weight, supporting gut health, minimizing stress, prioritizing sleep and ensuring adequate physical activity. We will explore this in more detail later on in the book.

Other Potential Causes of Autoimmunity

As with our hormonal health, we have the tools at our fingertips to balance our immune system and prevent autoimmunity. Effectively managing stress, eating as well as we possibly can, being mindful of medications, supporting our magical microbiomes and exercising regularly are easy-to-implement strategies and are all within our control.

STRESS

Stress is unavoidable in our fast-paced, modern lives, and it has been shown to play a large role in triggering autoimmunity.[19] In fact, 80 per cent of individuals affected by an autoimmune disease confirmed that they experienced a stressful episode before they acquired an autoimmune condition.

Individuals who already suffered with a stress-associated disorder, such as post-traumatic stress disorder, were shown to have an increased risk of acquiring an autoimmune disease. Additionally, in individuals who already have an autoimmune condition, experiencing stress can also worsen autoimmunity symptoms. Learning to manage stress is vital for immune health, and we will explore how to do this effectively with evidence-based strategies explained in Part 2 of the book.

THE FOOD WE EAT

Diet can also increase our risk of acquiring an autoimmune disease, and the typical Western diet – which is high in energy (i.e. calories) and in the consumption of ultra-processed foods while being low in nutrients – has been shown to increase the risk of autoimmunity. This type of diet is an environmental trigger in people who have an increased genetic risk as it increases inflammation that wreaks havoc on our immune health.[20]

Eating an ultra-processed diet that is high in sugars and fat and low in nutrients can increase our risk of obesity and result in significant weight gain. Body mass index (BMI) is a commonly used body measurement tool, and it is associated with a possible increased risk of certain autoimmune diseases, which may be partly due to chronic inflammation and a dysregulated immune system caused by obesity. However, it should be highlighted that BMI is often viewed as a controversial screening tool because it does not differentiate between fat and muscle mass composition, which both have significant impacts on our immune system as well as inflammatory status.

> Approximately **75 per cent** of individuals with an autoimmune disease believe that nutrition and food play a significant part in their disease.

Consuming an ultra-processed and nutrient-devoid diet can indirectly affect autoimmunity risk due to the related comorbid disorders, such as obesity, metabolic dysregulation and inadequate blood-sugar control, that may occur from eating this way.[21]

This type of diet can also significantly impact the health of our gut microbiome and gut lining, and this is a huge issue as we know approximately 70–80 per cent of our immune cells are in our gut.[22] Research indicates that insufficient diversity of beneficial gut bacteria can put you at a greater risk of autoimmunity with poorer outcomes. Individuals who have an autoimmune disease nearly all have dysbiosis, which is an imbalance of the gut bacteria, and this greatly impacts immune function while increasing inflammation. In turn, this then further increases the risk of acquiring an autoimmune disorder in those individuals who are most at risk.

The condition 'leaky gut' is also regularly seen in individuals with an autoimmune condition.[23] For people with an increased risk of autoimmunity, maintaining diversity and balance of the gut microbiome is essential, as is ensuring a healthy gut lining so that toxins and undigested food particles cannot enter the bloodstream. If they do, they can create significant issues for the immune system leading to damaging inflammation. By keeping our gut health in tip-top condition, we may be able to put a stop to autoimmunity progressing, even if we are at a higher genetic risk of acquiring an autoimmune disease.

We will explore the role of gut health in greater detail in Chapter 5 and we will also look at how and what we should eat for optimal gut health and immune function in Part 2 of the book.

AGEING

Ageing is something we cannot avoid, and unfortunately, it is associated with a gradual decline of the immune system. This is referred to as 'immunosenescence' and it can lead to an increased risk of acquiring an autoimmune disease, infection, increased inflammation and experiencing a poorer response to vaccines. Why this happens is not fully known yet, but one possible reason is the shrinking of our thymus that occurs after puberty. This means we lose the ability to produce new T cells, and as we age, we may not be able to respond to immune issues as efficiently as a younger individual can. Therefore, as we get older, looking after our immune system is essential to reduce our risk of infection and autoimmunity.

INFECTIONS

Numerous infections can trigger autoimmunity, with rubella, hepatitis A, hepatitis C, herpes, cytomegalovirus (another herpes virus), parvovirus B19, human T cell leukaemia virus type 1 and the Epstein–Barr virus all shown to have a role.[24]

Recent research suggests that the SARS-CoV-2 infection may trigger or exacerbate autoimmune conditions such as Guillain–Barré syndrome and antiphospholipid syndrome, among others.[25] This may occur due to the infection 'switching on' our self-reactive immune cells.

> **The Epstein–Barr** virus causes glandular fever, also known as infectious mononucleosis or mono. Glandular fever is most common in people aged 15–24, although cases have been reported across all age groups.[26] Studies show that over 95 per cent of adults worldwide have been infected with the Epstein–Barr virus at some point in their lives.[27]

Summary

Autoimmunity occurs when our immune system begins to attack our healthy cells, tissues and organs, leading to autoimmune disease. At present, researchers believe there are between 80 and 150 autoimmune disorders. While a cure for autoimmune disease is not yet available, many of these conditions can be managed effectively with various holistic approaches, such as consuming a nutrient-rich diet, managing body weight, ensuring we get sufficient sleep, engaging in regular physical activity, reducing chronic stress in our lives and spending time with friends to promote mental well-being, all of which allows individuals to live healthy and fulfilling lives.

CHAPTER 3

Allergies and Infections

Allergies

Allergies are on the rise, and in Europe, allergies are viewed as the most common chronic disease: 20 per cent of individuals who suffer from an allergy have a life-threatening allergy as well as experience significant and life-altering anxiety daily.[1]

As in autoimmune disease, allergies result from an imbalanced immune system and inappropriate immune response. An allergy can occur when the body changes its normal immune response to an allergen, and these altered immune responses are highly specific as they are adaptive immune responses. So, for example, an individual may have an allergy to one antibiotic but can safely take a different antibiotic. However, there are allergies that are known as 'contact' allergies, and these are different as it is our lymphocyte cells and macrophages (white blood cells that detect, engulf and destroy bacteria and other harmful organisms) that are overreacting to a metal or washing powder, for example. In most other allergies it is the antibody response that overreacts.

Allergies are also believed to be a result of lifestyle due to increased toxins, chemical exposure, pollution, changes in diet and nutrition, vitamin D deficiency, poor gut health and bacterial diversity, which impact how our immune systems react to certain harmless environmental exposures. As yet, we don't have the exact answers as to why allergies are on the rise, but they appear to run in families; therefore, we are aware that genetic predisposition does play a role. If either parent has an allergy, their child is more at risk of also developing it.

> **The atopic march** is a pattern that is described clinically in those with atopic disease, beginning as atopic dermatitis or eczema in infancy, then developing into allergic rhinitis, known as hay fever, and finally asthma later in childhood.[2]

Let's look at some of these allergies in more detail.

ECZEMA

Eczema, also known as atopic dermatitis, is a condition where the skin is incredibly dry and itchy. It can also make the skin appear cracked, crusty, scaly or thickened. It may present as red, white, purple or grey, or lighter or darker than the skin around it depending on your skin tone, and the skin may also blister or bleed. Eczema can appear in different areas of the body, but it is common on the elbows, knees and hands, and in babies and young children it may also appear on the face. This disease almost always starts before a child is five years old, although it can occur in individuals of any age: eczema affects about 20 per cent of children and up to 10 per cent of adults.[3] It is not fully known what causes eczema, but you are at an increased risk if one or both of your parents have the condition or if you or a close family member have asthma or hay fever.

Indoor irritants, such as the house dust mite, can trigger eczema,

ALLERGIES AND INFECTIONS

and the majority of people with eczema will find that they are sensitive to the house dust mite that thrives in warm damp places, including their bedding. While we cannot eliminate house dust mites completely, there are things we can do to limit the impact they may have on our skin, such as washing bedding at a high temperature (at least 60°C) as this can kill the house dust mites. It is also sensible to encase pillows and mattresses.

Animals can trigger allergic reactions in some with asthma or hay fever, and sadly, the saliva and fur of our beloved pets could irritate or worsen eczema. If you have pets and are experiencing eczema, it may be a good idea to avoid having them in your bedroom, particularly on your bed. Also, as much as we love cuddling our pets, if you are experiencing eczema symptoms, refrain from sitting on the sofa with them in very close contact.

Irritants such as indoor and outdoor mould can also be a problem. A damp and warm environment encourages mould, so it is important to ventilate rooms such as the bathroom and kitchen daily, as this will help to prevent a build-up of mould. Putting food waste out daily will also help prevent mould spores building up. Another useful tip is to wear gloves when gardening, and keeping compost heaps covered may also help. Moulds tend to be active in the spring and summer months and dormant in the winter months; autumn is the mould-sporing season and during this time you may find you have a flare-up.[4]

Eczema symptoms tend to get better as a child gets older, though there also tend to be times when symptoms worsen and a flare-up may be experienced, and times when the symptoms improve and go into remission. This irritating skin condition can be made worse by certain factors, including coming into contact with an allergen or irritant such as soap, washing detergent, pets, some fabrics, pollen or certain foods. Additionally, heat or changes in temperature, skin infections like a staph infection, stress and hormonal changes, such as those experienced during pregnancy, can all play a role in worsening eczema symptoms.[5]

One of the main issues with eczema is the desire to itch, but when this happens you are at an increased risk of infection. I have seen this happen first-hand with my daughter, who would scratch her skin intensely and most often when she was unaware during sleep. This resulted in her skin becoming infected and the eczema spreading, leading to her needing to be prescribed antibiotic cream.

> It is important to use topical ointments and creams, but note that emollients and paraffin-based treatments are **flammable**. You must avoid smoking, sources of ignition such as candles, open or wood-burning fires, gas cookers and naked flames when applying topical treatments to yourself or a child.

Skin, when it is healthy, is a brilliantly effective barrier against environmental stressors; however, in children with eczema, if food enters into the skin barrier, this may sensitize them towards a food allergy. In a small number of children, eczema is the result of sensitization to foods, most frequently cow's milk, eggs, peanuts, wheat, nuts and fish.[6] Keeping the skin moist is vital as this will limit the skin cracking, making it harder for allergens to enter. In turn, this will reduce the risk of a child affected by atopic dermatitis developing a food allergy.

Some children do appear to grow out of the condition, although it may return in adolescence; however, for half of those who possess the filaggrin mutation (a genetic change in the filaggrin gene which can cause a weakened skin barrier, leading to increased water loss and permeability to allergens and irritants), eczema is a lifelong disease.

HAY FEVER

Hay fever, also known as allergic rhinitis, is a condition which affects the inside of the nose and is caused by an allergen to which the immune system then responds inappropriately. It is a global health concern affecting approximately 400 million people worldwide.[7]

This condition is associated with symptoms of nasal congestion, sneezing and itching of the eyes, nose and throat. Sufferers are also likely to experience allergic conjunctivitis (pink eye or red eye), which causes redness and swelling of the eye.[8] One study showed that 64.1 per cent of patients with conjunctivitis also reported rhinitis, and 51.1 per cent of patients with rhinitis also suffered from conjunctivitis.[9]

Other symptoms of hay fever include:

- headaches
- blocked sinuses that may cause facial pain
- loss of smell and taste
- fatigue
- mucus running down the back of the throat, known as post-nasal drip
- feeling generally unwell due to the inflammatory nature of hay fever.

> Rates of **hay fever** have increased significantly over the last four decades.[10]

The number of adult hay fever sufferers is estimated to be 23 to 30 per cent of the population in Europe and 26 per cent in the UK.

In the United States, an estimated 15 per cent of the population, approximately 50 million individuals, are believed to be affected by allergic rhinitis.[11] While prevalence of the condition has soared over the last 40 years, we do not fully know why; it is thought that increasing recognition of the condition may be one reason, but it could also be a result of increasing urbanization, environmental pollutants and a wider trend of increasing prevalence of allergic diseases.

Hay fever has a peak incidence during the second to fourth decade of life, with most patients developing symptoms before the age of 20.[12] Before adolescence, boys have an increased incidence of the condition, but this reverses post-adolescence.[13] Family history is also key as there is an evident genetic link; in fact, research has confirmed that identical twins show 45 to 60 per cent concordance, while non-identical twins show 25 per cent.[14]

> **Concordance** refers to the extent to which a pair of individuals (often twins) share a particular trait or characteristic.

Hay fever has traditionally been categorized as seasonal or perennial (all year), depending on the temporal pattern of symptoms. If you suffer from hay fever, it is advisable to consider your home and work environment to identify if there are any triggers present that may be causing you symptoms, such as dust, fumes and other pollutants. Irritants such as smoke and traffic pollution can worsen hay fever and should be avoided where possible.

If your hay fever is triggered by pets, then it is a good idea to limit pets going into the bedroom and lying on the bed, and wash clothes at higher temperatures. Children and teenagers can be particularly affected by both active and passive exposure to second-hand smoking, leading to an increased risk of allergic diseases such as hay fever, eczema and food allergy.[15] Also, many drugs can cause or worsen rhinitis symptoms, including alpha and beta blockers, non-steroidal anti-inflammatory drugs, aspirin, antihypertensives, oral contraceptives and topical sympathomimetics.[16]

ASTHMA

Asthma is the most common chronic illness in children in the UK, and approximately 70 per cent of children who suffer with eczema go on to develop asthma.[17] In addition, research has shown that overweight or obese children are at greater risk of asthma and this is a main cause of hospitalization in children.[18] We will discuss body weight in Chapter 4 as it plays an incredibly important role in healthy immunity.

Asthma is characterized by inflammation leading to bronchoconstriction, which is when the muscles in the airways tighten, narrowing them and making it hard to breathe; oedema (swelling); and increased mucous production in the airways. Interestingly, the condition is more prevalent in boys in the first decade of life; however, after puberty and in the second decade of life, research indicates that asthma is more prevalent in young women.[19] A reason for this may be due to boys under the age of ten having a smaller airway size compared with girls of the same age, height and weight.[20] Asthma is considered a chronic disease of childhood, but there are periods of time during which the disease can go into remission or resolve altogether.

When symptoms of asthma worsen, this is known as an asthma attack. Some asthma sufferers have worse symptoms at night or during exercise, when they have a cold or during changes in the weather. Other triggers can include dust, smoke, fumes, grass and tree pollen, animal fur and feathers, strong soaps and perfume.

The most common symptoms of asthma include:

- a persistent cough, especially at night
- wheezing when exhaling and sometimes when inhaling
- shortness of breath or difficulty breathing, sometimes even when resting
- chest tightness, making it difficult to breathe deeply.

The genetics of asthma is complex, with multiple genes believed to contribute to asthma. Rapidly changing technology is continuing to increase our current understanding of the genetic risk factors for asthma development, and genome-wide association studies (GWAS) have improved our understanding of asthma susceptibility genes. A GWAS is a research approach used to identify genomic variants that are statistically associated with a risk for a disease or a specific trait. GWAS have identified over 100 different genes that influence the likelihood that an individual will get asthma. However, genetics is a small part of the picture as asthma is a complex condition influenced by both genetic and environmental factors, so further research in this area is needed.

> **Maternal asthma** is more strongly associated with childhood asthma development, and maternal tobacco smoking during pregnancy has been confirmed to increase the risk of childhood asthma.[21]

As we will see shortly when we look at the risk of food allergy in children, maternal diet in pregnancy is a risk factor in asthma. A high sugar intake during pregnancy has been associated with a greater risk of asthma in children.[22] However, studies have demonstrated that maternal diets that are higher in vitamin E, zinc and polyunsaturated fatty acids may be protective against the development of childhood asthma.[23]

In addition, pre-eclampsia, a condition that some women may experience in pregnancy, and Caesarean section (C-section) delivery have been shown to contribute to an increased risk of childhood asthma development.[24] This is certainly not to say that if you have a C-section, your child will definitely have asthma; in fact, both my children were born by C-section and neither has asthma. Low birth weight has also been associated with mid-childhood asthma diagnosis, with symptoms continuing into adult life.[25]

> **Gene–environment interactions** have been reported to be key for the development of childhood asthma.[26]

In adults, asthma is a common condition, with most recent figures showing asthma affecting an estimated 262 million adults worldwide in 2019 and causing 455,000 deaths.[27] It is often under-diagnosed and under-treated, particularly in low- and middle-income countries. Individuals with under-treated asthma may experience disturbed sleep, fatigue and poor concentration, and due to their condition, they and their families may need to be absent from school and work and this may impact the family financially.

While asthma cannot be cured, the most common treatment is using an inhaler, which delivers medication straight to the lungs. This can help to manage the disease and allow individuals to enjoy a normal, healthy and active life. Some people with asthma may find they need to use their inhaler daily, though treatment will depend on the frequency of symptoms.

FOOD ALLERGY

Food allergy is a major health issue, and its prevalence has increased significantly in the last 20 years, especially in Westernized developed countries.[28] Developing countries are showing similar patterns as their economies grow and their populations embrace a more Westernized lifestyle.[29] At present, overall food allergy prevalence is estimated to be 5 per cent in adults and 8 per cent in children.[30]

> In Europe **14 foods** (celery, cereals containing gluten, crustaceans, eggs, fish, lupin, milk, molluscs, mustard, peanuts, sesame, soybeans, sulphur dioxide and sulphites, and tree nuts) have been classified as major allergens, while in the US, there are believed to be **8 major food allergens** (milk, eggs, fish, crustacean shellfish, tree nuts, peanuts, wheat and soybeans).[31] These are commonly referred to as the 'Big 8' and are thought to account for 90 per cent of the food allergies.

When I had my first child, I was confused by the guidance I had previously heard from friends and family. I had been told that it was best to avoid giving young children (from weaning age up to approximately 12 months) the foods that most often trigger allergies, such as cow's milk, eggs, peanuts, fish and soya. However, research now suggests that *not* feeding children these foods could have resulted in an increase in food allergies. Furthermore, by not initially feeding certain foods but then incorporating them into the diet when older, this could have the unexpected result of triggering allergies.[32] The current advice is to introduce a varied diet at approximately six months of age while continuing, if you are able to, to breastfeed for a further six months after weaning. Breastmilk is easy for babies to digest and it also helps strengthen and balance their immune system.

What mums eat is key

Research has shown that maternal nutrition during pregnancy is key as it can impact baby's immune development. Consuming a diet rich in fish, fruit and vegetables in addition to specific nutrients, such as fibre, omega-3 fatty acids, zinc, selenium and antioxidant vitamins, has been associated with a decreased risk of allergic disease in children.[33]

While many of these factors have direct effects on the immune system, there is increasing research that protective benefits may also occur because of the beneficial impact on the gut microbiome. In the first study of its kind, mothers' intakes of different fibre sub-types – soluble fibre, insoluble fibre, prebiotic fibre and resistant starch – and subsequent allergic disease in babies were analysed.[34] In this observational study, which included 639 mother–infant pairs (all infants had a family history of allergic disease), the researchers discovered that greater maternal dietary intakes of resistant starch were associated with decreased medically diagnosed infant wheeze. These findings were consistent with an earlier observational study confirming a protective relationship between maternal resistant starch dietary intake and reduced infant wheeze.[35]

SOLUBLE FIBRE foods: black beans, kidney beans, chickpeas, broccoli, Brussels sprouts, sweet potatoes, turnips, carrots, apples, apricots, avocados, peaches, pears, plums, figs, flaxseeds, sunflower seeds, hazelnuts and oats.

> **INSOLUBLE FIBRE foods:** whole grains, wheat bran, brown rice, nuts, asparagus, green beans, potatoes, berries, kiwi, spinach and cabbage.
> **PREBIOTIC FIBRE foods:** apples, bananas, cauliflower, chicory root, Jerusalem artichokes, onions, garlic, leeks, barley, oats, Konjac root (elephant yam), cocoa, flaxseeds and seaweed.
> **RESISTANT STARCH foods:** green (unripe) bananas, pinto beans, soybeans, chickpeas, lentils, brown rice, oats and high-carbohydrate foods such as potatoes, which are then left to cool to become rich in resistant starch.

Following a varied and nutritious diet with sufficient intake of fibre is essential for a developing baby's health, particularly prebiotic fibre as it 'feeds' the beneficial gut bacteria, allowing them to thrive and carry out their important roles in our bodies. Research has confirmed that children with food allergies are lacking in specific gut bacteria species that are essential in educating our regulatory T cells, or Tregs, to tolerate foods that may cause an allergy, as well as teaching them to tolerate environmental substances, such as pollen. These missing gut bacteria species also play a vital role in educating the immune system.

It is very clear that what mums-to-be eat before and during pregnancy is crucial. Studies have shown that high consumption of fast food (three times or more a week) and low fruit and vegetable consumption (three times or fewer a week) increase the risk of allergy.[36] Therefore, focus on consuming a nutritious diet with lots of variety, as this is essential to give your baby the best start in life.

IGE FOOD ALLERGY

A true food allergy causes an immune response involving immunoglobulin E (IgE) antibodies, which impacts numerous organs leading to adverse symptoms such as facial or throat swelling, hives, itching and digestive discomfort. Sadly, the allergic reaction can be life-threatening if anaphylaxis occurs. Several studies have reported IgE mediated food allergy (the most common type, triggered by the immune system producing the IgE antibody) to be a significant public health issue which affects approximately 3 to 10 per cent of adults and 8 per cent of children worldwide.[37]

Food allergy is very different to a food intolerance, as even though in food intolerance symptoms can appear quite quickly, these symptoms are frequently delayed by up to 48 hours and can persist for hours or in some cases days. The symptoms experienced in food intolerance are generally less serious, and an individual experiencing food intolerance may just experience digestive issues, whereas it is the occurrence of a specific immune response that determines if someone has a true food allergy.

Meanwhile, it is the digestive system that triggers a response in a suspected food intolerance, when the body is unable to break down a food or substance efficiently or it responds to a food that you are sensitive to. An example of this is when the body is unable to break down lactose, which is a sugar found in dairy. If you are intolerant to a food, this can lead to unpleasant symptoms such as digestion issues, bloating, painful gas, constipation, diarrhoea and nausea. You may have an intolerance to a food due to a lack of the enzyme required to break it down; a chemical sensitivity to a food component – for example, caffeine; an adverse response to substances such as chemical additives, including preservatives, colouring and artificial sweeteners; or an increased sensitivity to a natural compound that occurs in a food, such as fructans, which are a type of carbohydrate.

Fructans are found in plant foods, such as wheat, barley, leeks, cabbage and onions, and can potentially cause irritable bowel syndrome (IBS) symptoms. These non-digestible carbohydrates are fermented by our gut bacteria, and this fermentation process then produces health-promoting short-chain fatty acids (SCFAs), which play an important role in supporting gut health as well as potentially overall health. Fructans are considered prebiotics as they promote the growth and activity of beneficial bacteria, such as bifidobacteria and lactobacilli.

If you suspect you may have a food intolerance, then I recommend keeping a food journal to note down when exactly you get symptoms, what type of symptoms you experience and the exact food or foods you ate prior to getting symptoms. If you are still unsure of the food that is causing you issues, then I recommend following an elimination diet, which we will discuss in Part 2.

> **Allergies** are a symptom of **immune dysregulation** and **inflammation**, so it is important to focus on following a diverse, nutritious, anti-inflammatory eating plan to ensure optimal gut and immune health.

Infections

Infections are the result of harmful pathogens, such as bacteria, viruses, parasites and fungi, entering the body, then multiplying and causing havoc. Infectious diseases represent a major health problem worldwide both in terms of morbidity and mortality. Fortunately, in the UK we have routine vaccinations that protect against many of these infectious diseases.

Bacteria and viruses are the most common cause of infections, with viral infections, which are present on a pandemic scale, continuing to be a significant threat. Whereas antibiotics can manage infections caused by bacteria, there are comparatively few antiviral medications that have been developed to manage emerging infectious diseases caused by viruses.

In a viral infection, the interferon system is our first line of defence, and this powerful system aims to stop the virus infection spreading in the body. This system is very reliant on sufficient vitamin C intake, as well as manganese, which is a mineral. The immune system is unable to eliminate some of these infections permanently and the sneaky viruses can 'conceal' themselves in our cells. Here, they bide their time, waiting to be re-activated, which can then lead to recurrent attacks, such as in the herpes virus when cold sores reappear on the lips and mouth.

Why Men Are Affected More

Generally, women tend to have a stronger immune response so can often clear infections faster than men. Research on respiratory disease suggests that this could be due to the role that oestrogen and testosterone play. As we saw earlier, as women have two X chromosomes, this may provide increased immunity to combat certain infections, such as what appeared to occur with Covid-19.

Why Do People Respond to Infections Differently?

Some people experience more gastrointestinal bacterial infections while other people experience more respiratory viral infections. A complex combination of pathogen, genetic and environmental factors all play a significant role in determining both susceptibility to particular pathogens and the course of the infection.[38]

As we saw with Covid-19, some people did not even know they were infected while tragically for others it was fatal. One study suggests that people who did not experience the worst symptoms may potentially have the 'right' balance of a type of immune white blood cells, known as macrophages. These cells are found in every tissue and are part of a group of cells called myeloid cells, which are fundamentally the 'guards' of our immune system. They are also healers and play an essential role in wound repair by heading to an injury to help the body to heal. These hard-working cells also fight potentially harmful invaders, gobbling them up and digesting anything that appears 'foreign' to the body, such as bacteria that could cause us harm. This attacking mode aids in maintaining our health; however, it also appears to be a factor in severe Covid-19 cases. Some data suggests that many Covid-19 deaths were a result of a hyper-immune response, with macrophages attacking not just the virus but also our bodies. This resulted in extreme and excessive inflammation that caused damage to organs such as the heart and lungs. A 2022 study conducted at Boston University's National Emerging Infectious Diseases Laboratories and Princeton University evaluated why this happened. The researchers investigated why some people became dangerously ill and why others didn't. By looking at lung tissue that appeared to combat SARS-CoV-2 efficiently or recover quickly from infection, they discovered a set of genes that determined whether immune cells would launch a balanced and capable defence or react uncontrollably and increase the risk of an individual becoming very ill and hospitalized.[39]

One symptom which presented in everyone I knew who had contracted Covid-19 was a fever. Even though having a fever can be uncomfortable it is a sign that the immune system is busy and working as it should. It is acceptable to allow a low-grade fever to resolve on its own, and recent research has shown that treating the fever with paracetamol to reduce it should be delayed, if possible. That being said, I think it is sensible to listen to your own body, so if you need to take medication to control a fever and make yourself more comfortable, do so.

Everyday Minor Infections

We are all different in how we respond to having an infection as well as how we acquire infections in the first place. There are factors which increase our risk of infection that we have no control over, such as gender, genes, age and previous exposure to a pathogen.

Minor infections, such as cough or cold, are very common; however, they can impact significantly on an economic level through lost productivity. A 2024 report by the Office of Health Economics (OHE) estimated the annual cost of all respiratory infections to UK businesses as £44 billion. While we can't avoid germs and infections entirely, there are factors that we can focus on improving that are in our control.

Nutrition and diet are key as a nutrient-deficient diet can lead to compromised immune health and impact our antimicrobial defences. We need to ensure sufficient intake of protein and omega-3 fatty acids as these will provide the resources required to fight infections. Even minor vitamin and mineral deficiencies can place you at a greater risk of acquiring an infection.[40] Stress management, physical activity, sleep and ensuring sufficient exposure to sunlight are also essential to immune health and fighting infections. We will look at how we can improve these areas of health in Part 2 of the book.

> **Two to four respiratory infections** per year is generally considered typical for adults, according to the NHS. However, for individuals who have certain conditions, such as cancer or heart disease, or those who have to take medication that impacts the immune system, it is harder to avoid everyday infections.

It is also important to highlight that good hygiene habits and vaccinations can help to reduce our risk of acquiring an infection. Ensuring basic hygiene is vital as potentially harmful pathogens enter through the skin barrier or openings in the body, such as the nose, mouth, eyes or gastrointestinal and urogenital tracts. Washing your hands and using tissues are key to avoiding several minor infections and protecting others. Public health is the responsibility of all of us as it impacts how infections are spread.

Hydration is another important factor to consider as adequate hydration has been associated with decreased risk of infection. It ensures your mucus membranes are moist, and this helps the barrier defend against infection as well as facilitates the flow of lymph and blood. This enables the immune cells to reach all areas of the body so they can carry out their important surveillance role, identifying and neutralizing harmful invaders and abnormal cells. If you don't consume a sufficient amount of fluids during an infection, this may impact how efficiently you recover and bounce back from the illness. It is crucial to continue to drink the recommended 1.5 to 2 litres of water a day if you can, or mix intake up by including soups, herbal teas or smoothies.

Ensuring enough rest is vital for getting back to full health. As we have seen, everyone responds differently to infections, but make sure you are resting your mind as well as your body because worrying about being ill or missing work can use up a lot of energy. Be kind to yourself and allow yourself time to recover and heal.

Summary

Allergies are on the rise on a global scale and are now seen as the most common chronic disease. As we saw with autoimmune disease, allergies are the result of an imbalanced immune system and an inappropriate immune response. Infectious diseases are also a major health concern affecting people worldwide. Infections occur when pathogens, such as bacteria, viruses, parasites or fungi, enter the body. Bacteria and viruses are the most common cause of infections. While many bacterial infections can be treated with antibiotics, there are comparatively fewer medications available to treat viral infections. So, we need our immune system working in tip-top condition to help us combat a viral infection. As with reducing our risk of autoimmune disease, a balanced immune system is essential to protect us against infections while also helping to prevent allergies.

CHAPTER 4

Immunometabolism

Immunometabolism is a fascinating field of research that explores the interactions between metabolic processes and the immune response. This close connection plays a key role in maintaining our health as metabolic changes in the immune system play an essential role in multiple diseases. When we talk about metabolism, we are referring to the chemical process that converts the food and drinks that we consume into energy. It is essentially the sum of all the chemical reactions happening in our body's cells to maintain life, powering everything from breathing to circulating blood, repairing damaged tissues, removing waste products, digestion and even thinking.

Our metabolism is also involved in maintaining the energy requirements of our immune system, therefore, these two systems are very much connected. An immune response demands a significant amount of energy, and our mitochondria (small organelles in our cells) help to convert the food and drinks we consume into energy by producing adenosine triphosphate (ATP). It is our mitochondria that help change immune cells swiftly into a metabolically active state so they can perform specific roles, including combating infection and fighting inflammation. This happens, for example, when we are ill and have a fever, and this results in a greater metabolic demand. Fever induction occurs at a high metabolic cost, such that only a 1°C rise in body temperature requires a 10 to 12.5 per cent increase in metabolic rate.[1] We need to look after our mighty mitochondria as if they are damaged this may incite an inflammatory response and lead to unwelcome inflammation.

At the same time as generating energy, our mitochondria generate oxidative stress (an imbalance between free radicals and antioxidants in the body that can lead to cell and tissue damage), which is a normal by-product of metabolism. This is why we need to maintain optimal antioxidant status, so we can combat oxidative stress effectively. Lifestyle is key in maintaining mitochondrial health as a nutrient-poor diet, pollution, smoking, stress and insufficient sleep can all impact our mitochondria. If our mitochondria are adversely affected, this can result in the damaged mitochondria releasing immune-cell signalling molecules called damage-associated molecular patterns (DAMPs) that turn on inflammation through the 'inflammasome'. The inflammasome are basically a security team for your body's cells and are vital for a healthy immune response to help you fight off infections and heal from injury. But when they are overactive or don't turn off properly, they can contribute to numerous inflammatory diseases. This happens because long-term, uncontrolled inflammation starts to damage healthy tissue.

Furthermore, when our mitochondria don't function as well as they should, it can lead to immune-associated disorders, poor energy levels, cognitive issues, pain, chronic inflammation, increased oxidative stress and accelerated ageing.

> **Immune–metabolic** relationships form the basis of life and are at the centre of many diseases including immune-mediated diseases, metabolic syndrome and cancer.[2]

The Danger of Poor Metabolic Health

A few years ago, a group of researchers from the University of North Carolina published a research paper that found prevalence of metabolic health in adults to be alarmingly low, even in normal-weight individuals, with only 12.2 per cent of adults in the United States being metabolically healthy.[3] Research confirms that a significant number of adults are suffering from impaired blood-sugar control, high blood pressure and an undesirably sized waist measurement.

The blood-sugar roller coaster that many individuals experience on a continual daily basis can cause significant issues for immune health, including:

- increased inflammageing (a long-term, low-grade inflammation that develops with advanced age)
- production of advanced glycaemic end products (AGEs) that disrupt how immune cells work and promote further inflammation
- disruption of epigenetic methylation, which can lead to accelerated ageing.

Focusing on reducing elevated blood-sugar levels is vital. We want to aim for stabilized, balanced blood-sugar levels and prevent our blood sugar from rising too high and too quicky, otherwise the hormone insulin then overcompensates and this leads to blood sugar dropping very quickly. If this happens, it can lead to some very unpleasant symptoms, such as feeling sweaty, lightheaded and shaky. Thus, it is imperative for health that we prevent this blood-sugar roller coaster from occurring.

On average, about two hours after eating, your blood sugar should drop back down to a near pre-meal level. However, this is a general guideline, and responses can vary based on factors like age, diet and overall health. Also, we all respond differently to different foods when it comes to blood-sugar responses – even identical twins can demonstrate significant variations when they eat the same foods. Why this happens may be influenced by several lifestyle factors, including diet, physical activity, sleep and stress, and these are in our control. Exercise, for example, plays a very significant role as it tells our body to free up sugar from its tissues and pass it into the blood to aid our physical activity.

Balancing our blood-sugar levels is vital for immune health, metabolic health, gut health and overall health. As we get older and age, we are more at risk of poorer blood-sugar control as our pancreas often functions at a lower level, thereby impacting insulin production. Blood-sugar control may also be affected as we age, because we may engage in less exercise and movement. Therefore, managing and focusing on balancing our blood-sugar levels is even more important as we get older.

One study, which included older people, confirmed that walking at a moderate pace for 15 minutes after each meal was as beneficial at lowering blood sugar over a 24-hour period as walking for 45 minutes in one go.[4] Even including moderate-pace walking for 15 minutes while you do your shopping counts. Regular, weight-bearing exercise such as walking also helps support lean muscle mass, which aids in reducing blood sugar after eating.

When it comes to the food we eat, carbohydrates have the greatest impact on blood sugar, and the quality of carbohydrate is very important to consider. We want to focus on carbohydrates that have been minimally processed, such as whole grains, legumes (including chickpeas, beans and lentils), vegetables, fruit, nuts and seeds. These wholefoods are rich in fibre, which helps to prevent blood-sugar spikes, and they 'feed' beneficial gut bacteria that help regulate blood-sugar levels.

> Look for a minimum of **1g of fibre** for every 10g of carbs on food labels.

Reducing and limiting added sugar is key. Foods that are high in added sugars include cakes, biscuits and sweets, but added sugar is hidden in many foods – even bread has been found to contain sugar. It is vital to read the labels carefully as sugar has so many different names, such as glucose, sucrose, fructose, maltose and high-fructose corn syrup. Some types of sugar may sound healthy, such as agave nectar, brown rice syrup or maple syrup, but these still need to be recognized as sugar and kept to a maximum of 10 per cent of daily energy intake. So, for example, if you eat a 2,000-calorie diet, your added sugar intake needs to be kept to 200 calories or less.

There are many non-nutritive sweeteners available that are low in energy and are used as a sugar substitute. While these have been deemed safe to include in our diet by the European Food Safety Authority (EFSA), they can affect how our body handles sugar and can actually cause blood-sugar spikes. Research has also confirmed that they can promote cravings for sweet foods as well as lead to an increase in appetite and impact metabolism, weight gain and obesity. Paradoxically, non-caloric artificial sweeteners were introduced primarily to prevent metabolic syndrome (a group of health conditions that affect the heart or vessels and puts you at increased risk of type 2 diabetes), but unfortunately, they may promote dysbiosis (an imbalance in our gut microbiota) and glucose intolerance, resulting in the negative metabolic effects that they were intended to prevent.[5] Human studies have demonstrated that artificial sweeteners can have an adverse impact on blood glucose due to their potential effect on our beneficial gut microbes. One artificial sweetener, aspartame, was shown to increase the number of certain bacterial strains that are associated with metabolic disease, which we know can increase type 2 diabetes and heart disease risk.

> **Protein intake** is key as it helps to stabilize blood sugar. Eat the protein in your meal first as this will be even more effective at balancing blood-sugar levels.
>
> **Vinegar** has also been shown to help manage blood-sugar levels.[6] Apple cider vinegar is a great addition to include in your diet.

Suboptimal metabolic health can lead to conditions such as type 2 diabetes, heart disease and stroke, and can also affect immune health in numerous ways, including:

- increased risk of autoimmunity
- increased allergy risk
- decreased protection against infections
- reduced vaccine response
- how our immune organs function
- accelerated ageing of our immune system
- influencing immune rejuvenation
- inhibiting new immune cells from being produced.

OBESITY AND METABOLIC HEALTH

It is very clear that being overweight or obese can also have a significant impact on our metabolic health as well as our immunity. In turn, supporting our metabolic health can help promote immune health. An abundance of research has confirmed the significant role that nutrition, diet and lifestyle play in metabolic health. Unfortunately, modern diets are rich in excessive saturated fat, processed carbohydrates and salt while being deficient in fibre, vitamins and minerals, and these diets are a leading cause of the emergence of obesity-associated chronic diseases, the majority of which are linked to chronic inflammation.[7]

> **Overnutrition** has been found to increase susceptibility to the development of inflammatory diseases, autoimmune diseases and cancer.[8]

The escalating global increase in obesity, also referred to as 'globesity', represents one of the most serious public health challenges for societies and healthcare systems.[9] Obesity is associated with numerous other health conditions, and it also alters the communication between our fat cells and immune system. This may lead to an increased risk of developing an inflammatory disorder, metabolic issues, different cancers and infections, and individuals may experience a poorer response to vaccines.

Body composition, defined as what our body mass consists of – e.g. muscle, fat, bone, organs and water – is a key factor to consider when it comes to both metabolic health and immune health.

> **Fat and muscle** play a vital part in your risk of developing a long-term inflammatory disorder or an infection, and muscle prevents against several of the most common inflammatory health disorders.

In the past, fat has been poorly understood with many negative connotations; however, it is now acknowledged as an organ in its own right due to the role it plays in our body. Fat plays a fundamental role in regulating immunity and balancing inflammation, and white adipose tissue has been confirmed to play a critical role, not only as an energy store but as an important endocrine organ.[10] We need fat to survive: it makes hormones, insulates us, protects our organs and makes up a whopping 50 per cent of our brains. However, when we consume too many calories, this extra energy is stored away in our fat cells, and when we reach and exceed our individual fat-storage limit, then it affects fat's ability to perform its immune-regulating role. Our fat cells are unable to store the surplus of energy and are impacted metabolically, becoming imbalanced, larger and potentially dysfunctional, which can lead to metabolic imbalances and an increased risk of a significant number of chronic health issues. When this happens, we gain more fat around our organs, which is immunologically imbalanced, and this results in increased impaired metabolic health and inflammation.

It is important to highlight that individuals can have poor metabolic health even if they are not overweight or obese, as they may have dangerous levels of visceral fat, which is the fat surrounding our organs. Therefore, muscle is key when it comes to our immune health, and it is also vital for a healthy metabolism and good blood-sugar control, as our muscle cells need more energy to sustain them compared with fat cells.[11]

How to Measure Body Composition

Body mass index (BMI) is an individual's weight (kilograms) divided by the square of their height (metres). While it is a straightforward tool, it is not an ideal screening method as it does not consider someone's fat distribution or overall body composition, such as how much muscle they have compared with fat.

The waist-to-hip ratio (WHR) screening tool may be a more preferable measurement of fat distribution, as it can help provide insight into an individual's overall health. Individuals who have more fat around their midsection compared with their hips may be at an increased risk of acquiring certain inflammatory disorders.

> **To calculate WHR:** divide your waist measurement by hip measurement – e.g. 28-inch waist divided by 38-inch hips = 0.74.
> *A healthy measurement is 0.85 or less in women and 0.9 or less in men.*

There is a third screening tool, which assesses an individual's waist-to-height ratio (WHtR) and this measures body fat distribution.

> **To calculate WHtR:** divide your waist measurement by height (both measured in the same unit) – e.g. 28-inch waist divided by 67-inch height (5 foot 7) = 0.42.
> *A healthy measurement is 0.5 or less for people under the age of 40, 0.5–0.6 for ages 40–50 and 0.6 for people over 50.*

To measure the percentage of lean muscle mass and fat mass, a dual-energy X-ray absorptiometry (DEXA) scan can be useful. Despite the scan not providing a totally accurate result, it can be helpful to give an approximate amount of how much muscle and fat an individual has. Women should aim to have a body fat level of around 28 per cent or less, and men should aim to have 20 per cent or less.

Fortunately, through appropriate nutrition, adequate physical activity and lifestyle modifications, we can improve our body composition, as we will discover in Part 2 of the book.

Summary

Immunometabolism is an exciting area of research that looks at the relationship and interactions between metabolic processes and the immune response. This close association plays an essential role in supporting our health as metabolic alterations in the immune system play an important part in numerous diseases.

Obesity has been confirmed to impact the communication between our fat cells and immune system, which may lead to a greater risk of developing metabolic issues, infections, inflammatory issues and cancer. However, normal-weight individuals can also have poor metabolic health as they may have dangerous levels of visceral fat, which is the fat surrounding our organs. Maintaining muscle is essential for immune health, a healthy metabolism and optimal blood-sugar control, and this can be achieved through nutrition, adequate exercise, sufficient sleep and managing stress effectively.

CHAPTER 5

The Importance of the Microbiomes

The Gut Microbiome

There is a significant amount of interaction between our gut microbiome and immune system, which isn't surprising when you consider that almost 80 per cent of our immune system is in our gut.

When we talk about the gut microbiome, we are referring to the microbes living in our gut along with their genes. Microbes are tiny organisms that can only be seen through a microscope, and the major groups of microorganisms are bacteria, viruses, fungi (yeasts and moulds), archaea, algae and protozoa. The microbiome, now known as the 'second brain', is made up of an incredible 100 trillion microbes that weigh over four pounds. Over millions of years, our gut microbes have changed as we as humans have evolved, influenced by the foods that we eat. We need to eat a diverse, nutritious diet so that we can 'feed' our beneficial gut microbes, and subsequently, they can carry out their vital functions in our body, including:

- regulating our metabolism and extracting energy from our food
- helping to manage body weight and regulate appetite
- supporting our nervous system, brain and mental health through a communication network called the gut–brain axis

- making hormones and neurotransmitters, which are brain chemicals
- manufacturing vitamins, such as vitamins B and K
- producing molecules called short-chain fatty acids (SCFAs) that support the gut barrier, helping to reduce the risk of 'leaky gut'
- aiding gut function and movement
- metabolizing medications
- deactivating toxins
- educating and training our immune system.

Our gut microbes also play an essential role in supporting our immunity. These mighty microbes interact with our immune cells, stimulating and modulating their responses. Ultimately, they are helping us maintain a healthy and balanced immune system. Changes in our gut microbes can have a huge impact on the body's T helper cells, which help support your immune system's response to potentially harmful pathogens. Unfortunately, these industrious cells can remain in 'overdrive', which means the immune response carries on without stopping, and this is what leads to immune function issues and increases your risk of autoimmune disease.

Over the last 15 years, studies have confirmed that the gut microbiome plays a vital role in shaping the immune system and impacting our health. Further research has suggested that the increase in autoimmunity may be due to the relationship between our gut microbes and body being disrupted. Thus, it is essential that we look after our microbes as they are involved in so many different areas of health. In fact, they are involved in most, if not all, of the body's biological processes.

Beneficial gut bacteria species influence both innate and acquired immunity. Our gut microbiota interacts with the gut-associated lymphoid tissue (GALT), which as we know houses a significant portion of the body's immune cells, to modulate immune responses. From birth, our gut bacteria train and educate our immune system. You may have heard about a concept known as the 'hygiene hypothesis', which suggests that decreased exposure to different microorganisms in early childhood may increase the risk of developing allergic and autoimmune diseases. This is because a lack of exposure to germs in early life can disrupt the normal development of the immune system, which then may result in the immune system overreacting to harmless substances.

> **Microbes** are types of microorganisms, including bacteria, viruses, fungi (yeasts and moulds), algae, archaea and protozoa.

Genetics, diet and lifestyle choices have the most significant impact on shaping the gut microbiome. As we know, we cannot change the genes we have been given, but we can change the make-up of the different species of bacteria through appropriate diet and lifestyle modifications. Diversity is essential as different bacteria play different roles in maintaining our health. Some bacteria help us digest food and absorb nutrients while other bacteria support our immune system and others help protect against harmful pathogens. To ensure sufficient diversity in our gut microbiota we need to focus on consuming a varied diet, including lots of different plant foods as well as daily servings of fermented foods, such as live natural yoghurt, cheese, miso, tofu, kefir and sauerkraut.

Unfortunately, in the Western world, due to the ultra-processed diet that many people eat, and also due to antibiotic use, many of the beneficial gut bacteria that evolved with us over millions of years don't exist any more, or if they do, they are present in a significantly lesser quantity. The lack of these bacteria impacts our immune health, so our immune system may not function as well as it could. However, we are able to re-establish many of these microbes through appropriate diet and lifestyle changes, which will help us combat infections effectively, balance an overactive immune system and reduce allergy risk. It really is up to us.

Our gut microbiota has considerable plasticity (adaptability) and can change significantly in response to diet. This is a key modifiable factor influencing the composition of the gut microbiota, albeit these changes appear to be temporary.[1] Therefore, while diet can promote a change in the gut microbiota, whether prolonged dietary changes can lead to permanent alterations in the gut microbiota is currently unknown due to the lack of long-term human dietary interventions or long-term follow-ups of short-term dietary interventions.

Also, if you have ever had a course of antibiotics, it is very likely that a lot of your beneficial bacteria have been eradicated. Research has confirmed that certain antibiotics can lead to long-term alterations to the gut microbiota – even one single course of antibiotics has been reported to result in adverse changes in gut microbiota composition and diversity. It is not surprising that compared with our ancestors, who did not have access to antibiotics, we now only have a very small proportion of gut bacteria species.

Good Gut Health = Balanced Immunity

Our gut microbiome plays an essential role in our immunity, and the interaction between our microbiome and immune system is ultimately what maintains our health. Balancing our immune system is crucial in reducing our risk of allergies and autoimmunity and preventing chronic disease.

Dysbiosis and Leaky Gut

Immune-mediated and metabolic diseases are increasing on a global scale,[2] and it is becoming increasingly clear that our gut microbiota plays a significant role in the development of many, if not all, of these diseases.[3] Many of these conditions are associated with changes in gut microbiota composition and function.[4] This imbalance in our gut microbiota is known as dysbiosis, which is when the gut bacteria and gut microbiome become imbalanced and can result in some potentially very unpleasant symptoms. At present, it is not clear whether dysbiosis is a direct cause of disease or simply reflects disease-induced changes in the immune and metabolic systems. However, there are examples of alterations in the gut microbiota that occur before the onset of disease, such as in the autoimmune disorder type 1 diabetes[5] as well as in Parkinson's disease.[6] In addition, many infectious diseases have been shown to promote dysbiosis, including the SARS-CoV-2 infection, which has been associated with dysbiosis of the gut microbiota.[7]

> **Constipated? Diarrhoea? Bloated? Gas? Cramps? Reflux? Indigestion?**
>
> These are all signs that you might be lacking in beneficial bacteria and experiencing gut dysbiosis.

The most typical features of dysbiosis are a reduction in the diversity of the gut microbiota, a loss of beneficial microbiota or an overgrowth of harmful microbiota.

Significant changes to the gut microbiota can be brought about by macronutrient consumption and this may have a profound effect.

An example of this is consuming a diet that is high in simple sugars, which wreaks havoc on our gut barrier, leading to gut inflammation and adversely affecting our metabolism and immunity. Dysbiosis can lead to systemic inflammation that is associated with autoimmunity, and can cause the immune system to 'malfunction', triggering an autoimmune condition. Research conducted by the University of Arizona concluded that dysbiosis plays a role in both rheumatoid arthritis and multiple sclerosis (MS).

Dysbiosis can be caused by numerous different factors, including genetics, health status, lifestyle and environment; consuming a poor diet that is high in sugar and low in fibre; exposure to xenobiotics (antibiotics, drugs and food additives); and also hygiene.[8]

> **Dysbiosis** can compromise the gut barrier, resulting in tissues and organs being flooded with molecules from the diet and microbiota that can negatively impact our immune system and metabolism.

Dysbiosis may also impact how effectively messages are being transmitted through the gut–brain axis by increasing inflammation and causing our gut barrier to become more permeable. This disruption may also lead to a variety of other health issues, including altered brain function as well as several neurological and psychiatric disorders.

It can also lead to 'leaky gut' syndrome, a condition that allows anything inside your gut – such as food, protein, bacteria, parasites or yeast – to 'leak' into your body and head into the lymphoid tissue and immune cells in your intestines and into the bloodstream. The immune cells respond by producing cells known as T helper cells. When you start producing too many T helper cells, issues then occur; while they are essential for fighting infections, excessive production can lead to harmful autoimmune reactions and an increased risk of autoimmune disease.

Leaky gut occurs when the tight junctions of your intestinal wall or gut barrier loosen, which can allow harmful toxins, bacteria or undigested food to escape into the bloodstream. Our gut barrier's main role is to keep harmful invaders out, but when these junctions get loose, these unwanted invaders can enter and wreak havoc. Research confirms that nearly all individuals affected by autoimmunity also experience leaky gut syndrome, even if they are not experiencing gut issues and symptoms.[9] This illustrates the importance of maintaining sufficient and diverse beneficial bacteria in our guts, as it's these beneficial bacteria that help to strengthen our intestinal wall. If we don't have a strong intestinal wall and gut barrier, our immune system may mount an immune response when these undigested particles of food, toxins or pathogens enter the bloodstream, and this can result in some unpleasant symptoms, such as diarrhoea, painful gas, bloating and constipation. Leaky gut can also lead to impaired immunity, fatigue, IBS, low mood, skin issues, pain and allergy-type symptoms.

Leaky gut risk factors include:

- chronic dysbiosis
- poor diet
- toxins
- excessive alcohol consumption
- antibiotic use
- stress
- surgery
- food poisoning

- medications, such as non-steroidal anti-inflammatory drugs (NSAIDs)
- chronic infections
- parasite infections
- emotional distress

Focusing on restoring a balanced and healthy gut microbiome is key and has been shown to help prevent leaky gut. If you are experiencing leaky gut, research shows that by having a healthy gut microbiome, it is possible to reverse the condition. In the next chapter, we will discover how you can repair your gut.

In addition to dietary and lifestyle interventions, probiotics could help to restore the gut microbiota. Probiotics have become very popular for their potential role in modulating the gut microbiota, and there is compelling data on the efficacy and safety of several probiotics, including *Lactobacillus* spp., *Bifidobacterium* spp. and *Saccharomyces* spp. Other promising probiotics include *Roseburia* spp. and *Faecalibacterium* spp.[10] Research has confirmed the successful use of probiotics in treating various diseases, including ulcerative colitis, IBS, acute diarrhoea and antibiotic-induced diarrhoea. There is also evidence that probiotics may be effective in the treatment of metabolic, cardiovascular and neurological diseases. However, high-quality randomized controlled clinical trials are needed to better understand which strains, formulations and dosages are effective for which conditions.

Another strategy that could help to restore the gut microbiota is faecal microbiota transplantation (FMT), the process of transplanting stools from a healthy individual into the gut of a diseased individual for therapeutic purposes. Research has indicated that the microbiota community could be completely restored by FMT.

One infection, known as *Clostridioides difficile*, causes high morbidity and mortality, and FMT has been very effective for recurrent *Clostridioides difficile* infections, with cure rates exceeding 90 per cent. It may be recommended as an initial treatment as most individuals with *Clostridioides difficile* infection recover after a first FMT treatment. This therapy has also been used experimentally to treat other gastrointestinal disorders, such as ulcerative colitis, constipation, IBS, liver diseases and alcoholic hepatitis, and neurological diseases, such as MS and Parkinson's disease.

The 'Other' Microbiome

In addition to the gut microbiome, we have another microbiome, which is known as the oral microbiome. Our mouth has the second largest and diverse microbiota after the gut, harbouring 700 species of bacteria as well as yeasts, viruses and some protozoa.[11] A balanced oral microbiome, with a diverse community of beneficial bacteria, is essential for maintaining oral health and supporting our body's immune defences. In fact, our oral microbiome significantly impacts immunity and influences immune responses. It plays a vital role in training the immune system, particularly the innate and adaptive immune responses, and influences the development and function of immune cells, including T cells and B cells, which are crucial for fighting off infections.

A healthy oral microbiome can help to maintain the integrity of the mucosal barrier and prevent pathogens from entering the body, as well as influence the production of inflammatory cytokines and help to regulate the immune response to infections. It can even affect how the body responds to certain medications, potentially impacting their effectiveness. But if the oral microbiome is imbalanced, this can weaken the immune system's ability to fight off infections, increasing the risk of respiratory infections, oral thrush and other conditions. Research shows that oral bacteria can actually translocate to other parts of the body, potentially contributing to the development of chronic diseases, such as cardiovascular disease and type 2 diabetes.

In recent years, the association between oral microbiota and systemic disease has gained attention as poor oral health is associated with several health conditions. Our respiratory tract begins in the mouth and finishes in the lungs, so it is not a surprise that an overgrowth of the oral microbiome can lead to microbes being inhaled into our lungs. This can frequently result in infections, including pneumonia, which is a very serious disease, particularly in older individuals. Poor oral hygiene has also been associated with chronic obstructive pulmonary disease and poorer respiratory function and is associated with changes in the oral microbiome.

Unfortunately, as with our gut, oral dysbiosis can occur and this may lead to numerous health issues, including an increased risk of infections and a worsening of inflammatory conditions. It can also increase the risk of oral diseases like periodontitis and gingivitis.[12] Periodontitis, a chronic gum disease, has also been associated with other diseases and health complications such as cancer, neurogenerative disease, chronic kidney disease, cardiovascular diseases, respiratory health issues and adverse pregnancy outcomes, and an increased risk of autoimmune disorders, such as rheumatoid arthritis and inflammatory bowel disease. Chronic gum disease is one of the most common oral microbiome diseases, and this condition can damage the bone and tissues that support the teeth, potentially leading to tooth loss. This disease is the result of an overgrowth of the bacteria that are found in the gaps between your teeth and gums due to poor oral hygiene.

Gum disease promotes a strong inflammatory immune response, and we know that inflammation is how the body fights infections, resulting in the production of immune cells and chemical signals that tackle infection. However, we also know that too much inflammation is harmful, and some researchers believe that inflammation caused by gum disease could harm the cardiovascular system. Research has reported a significant link between gum disease and cardiovascular disease,[13] though this may be due to common risk factors, such as cardiovascular disease and gum disease more frequently found in smokers. Other research has suggested that the bacteria that is present in gum disease may actually travel to the heart, leading to infection. Research has also demonstrated that treating gum disease could reduce inflammation levels in the blood and significantly improve artery function.[14]

Chronic gum disease has also been linked with an increased cognitive decline in individuals with Alzheimer's disease. Since gum disease and Alzheimer's disease are both associated with ageing, it is difficult to determine whether there is a clear cause-and-effect relationship; however, in 2019, researchers discovered that the brains of individuals with Alzheimer's disease were colonized with *P. gingivalis*, which is one of the main bacteria that cause gum disease.[15] As with cardiovascular disease, the inflammation that occurs due to gum disease may be a driver of Alzheimer's disease in individuals who have poor oral health.

> Changes in **oral microbiota** composition may contribute to sensitization and the development of allergic reactions, including asthma and peanut allergies. There is also evidence that allergic reactions within the gut may contribute to alterations in oral microbiota composition.[16]

Research has also shown that oral bacteria can travel to the stomach and into the intestines. Generally, though, our oral microbes are not well suited to this environment and normally die out; in fact, scientists believe that more than 99 per cent of these microbes die as they pass through the acidic environment of the stomach and later the small intestine, which act as a barrier between the bacteria of the mouth and the gut. Although, if this barrier fails, this can result in the overgrowth of oral microbes in the gut that may potentially contribute to the onset or development of diseases, such as bowel cancer, rheumatoid arthritis and inflammatory bowel diseases.

Even in healthy individuals, low levels of bacteria usually located in the mouth are frequently found in stools, and it is unclear if these bacteria cross the barrier or if they are similar bacteria that originate in the gut. Over the last decade, one such species, called *Fusobacterium nucleatum*, has been strongly indicated as a potential contributor to colorectal cancer growth. Although *F. nucleatum* is normally found in the mouth, researchers have confirmed that increased numbers of it are found in the intestines of people with colorectal tumours compared with people without cancer. Researchers also found that *Fusobacterium* has a high affinity for malignant cancer cells, as the surface of cancer cells encourages the bacterium to tightly bind and invade the tumour. Numerous studies have now confirmed that *Fusobacterium* can colonize tumours throughout the gastrointestinal tract.[17]

How to Achieve Optimal Oral Microbiome Health

Certain factors that can impact the health of your oral microbiome include dental hygiene, diet, smoking and medications. A regular oral hygiene routine is imperative, and this involves brushing twice a day and flossing daily to eliminate plaque and decrease the incidence of cavities and gum disease. Implementing a regular, effective oral hygiene routine will help to improve and maintain the health of your oral microbiome by preventing the growth of harmful bacteria.

Regular dental check-ups and professional cleanings are also vital to help address any potential oral health issues. The NHS recommends that adults in England and Wales with good oral health should have a dental check-up at least once a year. However, individuals with a higher risk of dental problems may need to visit more frequently, potentially every six months. Children and young people under 18 are also generally recommended to have check-ups every six months. Similarly, in the US, the Centers for Disease Control and Prevention (CDC) recommends visiting the dentist once per year.

What we eat and drink is also an essential consideration as what we consume plays a vital role in maintaining optimal health of our oral microbiome. Sugar, fat and vitamin intake can all contribute to the balance of your oral microbiome. Alcohol can also affect the balance of your oral microbiome, and if you are a smoker, stopping smoking can significantly decrease your risk of gum disease as well as cancer. Fortunately, as with our gut microbiome, we have the tools to improve our oral microbiome and reduce our risk of diseases associated with it.

The next chapter will explain what we need to do to support our gut health, which in turn will help to ensure a strong, balanced and healthy immune system.

Summary

Almost 80 per cent of our immune system is in our gut, so there is a vast amount of interaction between our gut microbiome (the microbes living in our gut along with their genes) and immune system. Microbes are types of organisms, and the major groups of microorganisms are bacteria, viruses, fungi, archaea, algae and protozoa.

Along with the gut microbiome, we do have another microbiome: the oral microbiome. Our mouths have been reported to harbour 700 species of bacteria, viruses, yeasts and protozoa. What we eat and drink is extremely important as it has a huge impact on both our oral and gut microbiomes, which we shall learn more about in the next chapter.

PART 2

Evidence-Based Strategies For Improved Immunity

CHAPTER 6

The Good Gut Health Plan

Gut health plays a huge role in our immune health as well as in autoimmune healing and preventing allergies. To fully heal and balance the immune system, we need to heal the gut lining and focus on strengthening the gut barrier to reduce our risk of experiencing leaky gut. If we don't, then the immune response may not improve, and the issue will persist and potentially worsen. Therefore, if you are experiencing dysbiosis and/or leaky gut syndrome, we first need to focus on treating these conditions.

But how do you know if you have these conditions?

The following questionnaires will give you a good idea of if you are suffering from dysbiosis and/or leaky gut syndrome.

Questionnaire 1 – Dysbiosis
Score 1 point for every time you answer yes.
1. Do you experience stomach cramps regularly (at least once a week)?
2. Do you have diarrhoea, gas or bloating most days?
3. Do you have mucus or blood in your stools regularly (at least once a week)?
4. Do you suffer from long-term constipation?
5. Do you have regular stomach bugs?
6. Are you intolerant to fibrous foods (e.g. beans, lentils, wholewheat bread)?

7. Do you have any other food sensitivities?
8. Do you experience daily brain fog?
9. Is your breath 'bad' or smelly?
10. Is your energy low most days?
11. Do you suffer from anxiety?
12. Do you suffer from low mood or depression?
13. Have you taken a course of antibiotics more than three times in 12 months?
14. Have you taken daily antacids for more than one month?
15. Do you suffer from long-term congestion of the sinuses?
16. Have you experienced vaginal or anal itching?
17. When you travel do you suffer from traveller's diarrhoea?
18. Are you experiencing long-term stress?
19. Have you been diagnosed with acid reflux or heartburn?
20. Do you have fibromyalgia?
21. Do you have a vitamin D deficiency?
22. Do you have a diagnosed autoimmune condition?

Once you have answered this questionnaire, please add up all your yes answers and refer to the points system below.

15+ This high score suggests that you may be experiencing chronic and severe dysbiosis. The imbalance between beneficial bacteria and more harmful bacteria could be causing significant issues. You should make substantial modifications to your diet and lifestyle. This book will guide you on how to make these changes. In addition, you may wish to work with a dietician or qualified nutrition practitioner who can help you implement these changes.

9–14 You may be experiencing mild-moderate dysbiosis that may be causing issues. You should make modifications to your diet and lifestyle. Follow the guidance in this book to help you implement the necessary changes. To support your gut health and immune system further, check where you answered yes and focus on making changes in these areas.

0–8 Well done – it sounds like you have sufficient levels of beneficial bacteria and little or limited harmful bacteria, parasites or yeast. You seem to have good gut health. Your low score does not fully guarantee that you do not have dysbiosis, but if you do, it may be very mild. To support your gut health and immune system further, check where you answered yes and focus on making changes in these areas.

Questionnaire 2 – Leaky Gut
Score 1 point for every time you answer yes.
1. Did you answer yes to 9–22 questions in the dysbiosis questionnaire above?
2. Do you have a diagnosed autoimmune disease?
3. Do you have more than one food sensitivity (e.g. gluten, wheat, eggs, dairy, shellfish or eggs)?
4. Do you suffer from unmanaged chronic stress?

Once you have answered this questionnaire, please add up all your yes answers and refer to the points system below.

2–4 Your score suggests that you are likely suffering from leaky gut and your gut barrier is impaired. This could be causing you significant issues. You should make substantial modifications to your diet and lifestyle. Follow the advice provided in this book to help you achieve these required changes. In addition, you may wish to work with a dietician or qualified nutrition practitioner who can help you modify your diet and optimize your nutrition.

0–1 Your score suggests that you do not appear to be suffering from leaky gut. However, your low score does not fully guarantee that you do not have leaky gut, but you do not have the factors or conditions associated with it, such as a diagnosed autoimmune disease, food sensitivities or unmanaged chronic stress. To support your gut health and immune system further, check where you answered yes and focus on making changes in these areas.

It is evident from the increasing research that one of the most important factors for a healthy immune system is optimal gut health, so let's discover what we need to do to ensure our gut is as healthy and balanced as it can be.

The Good Gut Health Plan

Firstly, we need to repair our guts, and we can do this by following an easy, straightforward programme that involves two different stages.

> Helpful hint – before you start Stage 1, you may wish to keep a food journal for five to seven days so you can monitor any foods that cause any uncomfortable symptoms.

Stage 1 – Foods to Remove

This stage lasts between two to four weeks for most people, depending on the severity of their symptoms. Our aim is to focus on repairing, and the first step is to remove any foods, toxins or chemicals that you think may be causing your digestive issues or other symptoms. Foods that can cause gut issues include gluten, eggs, dairy, soy, shellfish and coffee. Coffee may increase the frequency of contractions throughout your gut. While caffeine is often seen as the reason why coffee may cause digestive issues, studies have shown that coffee acids may also play a role.

Remove the following from your diet for these first two to four weeks:

- **Gluten and refined grains**
- **Legumes** (beans, chickpeas, lentils) – These contain lectin (a protein), which may cause bloating, discomfort and increased gut permeability, and possibly drive autoimmune diseases
- **Dairy products**
- **Fibrous vegetables** (broccoli, Brussels sprouts, cabbage)
- **Alcohol**
- **Coffee** (if this causes digestive issues for you)

Fibrous vegetables can cause digestive issues for some people as the indigestible fibre that is fermented by gut bacteria produces gas that can lead to bloating, cramping and digestive discomfort. Some high-fibre veggies also contain specific sugars that are difficult to digest or are high in fermentable carbohydrates that can cause digestive issues for individuals with sensitive guts.

If you follow a vegan eating plan and you don't experience any digestive issues eating legumes, then you can reintroduce them after the initial two weeks as these are an important protein and fibre source for vegans or those following a plant-based diet. In addition, they are packed with essential vitamins, minerals and powerful plant compounds called phytochemicals or phytonutrients.

> **Coffee** for some people can cause unpleasant symptoms due to the caffeine as it is a stimulant and can encourage the release of cortisol and adrenaline, two hormones associated with stress. Studies confirm that genes play a significant role when it comes to caffeine intolerance. Some individuals can enjoy more coffee than others with no ill effects. However, if you feel anxious or jittery after drinking coffee, I recommend eliminating it during the first stage of this programme.

Stage 1 also recommends removing dietary chemicals as they are harmful to gut health. Dietary chemicals include preservatives, emulsifiers and artificial sweeteners. We also want to focus on limiting chemicals produced by our own bodies, such as excessive cortisol, a stress hormone. Chronic stress has a huge, adverse impact on gut health and significantly increases our risk of acquiring an autoimmune disease.

Stage 1 – Foods to Include

- **Protein** – High-quality protein sources are vital to include during this stage as they are essential for repairing the gut lining. Protein sources to include in your diet: wild salmon, sardines, mackerel, free-range or organic eggs, tofu, tempeh, nuts and seeds.

How much protein should we consume?

In the **UK**, the adult Reference Nutrient Intake (RNI) is **0.75g** per kg of body weight per day, which is approximately **45g** per day for women and **56g** for men aged 19 to 50. However, this does not account for several factors that may increase a person's protein requirements. The British Heart Foundation and the British Dietetic Association recognize that protein requirements can be increased for certain groups, such as older adults, athletes and active people, or those recovering from illness or injury.

In the **US**, the Dietary Reference Intake (DRI) is **0.8g** of protein per kg of body weight, which is **46g** per day for women and **56g** per day for men. This is based on a sedentary individual, so if you exercise or have an active lifestyle, you will require more.

Some recent research suggests that increasing protein to **30–40g** per meal may provide extra health benefits, such as helping to maximize protein synthesis and prevent a condition called sarcopenia, which is the loss of muscle mass that occurs with age.

- **Healthy fats** – Include foods rich in monounsaturated fat, such as avocados, olives, olive oil, nuts and seeds. Research also suggests that the medium-chain fatty acids (MCFAs) in coconut oil may be easier to digest than other fats and may help to improve gut health and leaky gut symptoms. Coconut oil consists of 90 per cent saturated fat; however, it is different from the saturated fat in animal fats as more than 50 per cent of the fats in coconut oil are MCFAs, including lauric acid, of which coconut oil is the greatest natural source.
- **Vegetables** – Veggies are my number-one go-to source of carbohydrates. Focus on including lots of different

veggies of different colours in your diet as this diversity will ensure you are consuming a wide variety of vitamins, minerals, fibre and phytonutrients, which are powerful plant compounds that have anti-inflammatory, antioxidant and antimicrobial properties, which benefit health. Diversity, when it comes to plant foods, is paramount for achieving and maintaining optimal gut health and immune health.
- **Herbs and spices** – These powerful foods all count when trying to increase your consumption of plant foods. Herbs and spices such as turmeric, chilli, garlic, basil and rosemary are all very high in a group of plant compounds called polyphenols that have several benefits on our health, including promoting good gut health by boosting growth of our 'good' gut bacteria while preventing harmful bacteria.

Stage 2 – Reintroduction

Once you have completed Stage 1 you can move on to Stage 2, which involves reintroducing the foods that were removed in Stage 1.

It is advisable to reintroduce each food gradually, one by one, and each food over three days. This is because if you experience any symptoms after you reintroduce a specific food, you can remove it, leave it for a couple of days, then move on to reintroducing a different food.

- **Gluten** – It may be helpful to begin with sourdough bread as the wild yeast and bacteria (lactobacilli) in the leaven is able to neutralize phytic acid, which makes it much easier to digest. You can then reintroduce other grains such as rye, which tends to be lower in gluten, then finally move on to reintroducing wheat.

- **Dairy** – When it comes to reintroducing dairy, I recommend first introducing live natural yoghurt, which is rich in probiotic bacteria and can benefit gut health. Then move on to cheese, then butter and finally milk – try to reintroduce these foods in this order.
- **Legumes** – If you avoided legumes for the first four weeks, then you can now reintroduce them in Stage 2. These foods, such as beans, chickpeas and lentils, are a very important plant protein source for individuals who follow a plant-based diet.
- **Coffee** – Some individuals can drink coffee with no adverse effects, but if you removed coffee in the first stage of the programme, you can reintroduce it in stage 2. Drinking coffee on an empty stomach may irritate your gut lining, so having something to eat first can help to prevent this. Or you may wish to try decaf coffee if you are sensitive to caffeine's stimulating effects. You will still get the amazing health benefits that the polyphenols (powerful plant compounds that have strong antioxidant and anti-inflammatory properties) in coffee provide without the digestive discomfort.

In Stage 2 also focus on including foods that are rich in:

- **Glutamine** – This is the most abundant amino acid (building block of protein) in our body, and it is essential for gut health. It is gut-healing and promotes immune-cell activity in the gut, which helps to prevent inflammation and infections. Foods high in glutamine include bone broth, chicken, fish, beans, beets, cabbage, spinach, lentils and tofu.
- **Probiotics** – These are the live bacteria found in fermented foods, such as live yoghurt, sauerkraut, cheese,

kimchi, miso and kefir, which can provide benefits to health, such as improving digestive health as well as immune health. Sauerkraut, kimchi, kefir and miso soup can all be homemade, and they work out a lot cheaper with more diverse bacteria than shop-bought alternatives.

I get asked a lot whether probiotic supplementation is a good idea. The main concern is that research in this area is still fairly limited and we aren't sure yet of which strains should definitely be taken and whether they are suitable for all individuals. However, some research does suggest they may be helpful and beneficial if you are very young, old or very ill.[1] For the average individual I would focus on increasing your intake of fermented foods that are naturally rich in probiotic bacteria, such as those listed above.

- **Prebiotics** – This is a type of fibre that provides 'fuel' for your beneficial gut bacteria. Importantly, I must highlight a common misconception – not all fibre is prebiotic. To be classed as a prebiotic, the fibre must not be absorbed in the gut, it must be able to be fermented by the gut bacteria, and it must promote the growth and activity of certain microbes to improve health.[2]

    Prebiotic fibre is super-important as it encourages our gut bacteria to produce a short-chain fatty acid (SCFA) called butyrate. This very significant SCFA is crucial for optimal gut health and provides numerous other health benefits, such as supporting immunity, relieving gastrointestinal conditions such as IBS, reducing inflammation and preventing diseases such as colon cancer and cardiovascular disease. Butyrate has also been shown to support brain health and enhance sleep.

PREBIOTIC FOOD SOURCES

FRUITS	VEGGIES	LEGUMES	NUTS AND SEEDS	OTHER FOODS
Apples	Artichokes	Black beans	Almonds	Chicory root
Avocado	Asparagus	Black-eyed peas	Cashews	Cocoa powder
Bananas	Cauliflower	Butter beans	Chia seeds	Dark chocolate (70 per cent cacao minimum)
Blueberries	Dandelion greens	Chickpeas	Flaxseeds	Garlic
Kiwi	Leeks	Kidney beans	Hazelnuts	Honey
Nectarines	Mushrooms	Lentils	Pistachios	Oats
Watermelon	Onions	Mung beans	Pumpkin seeds	Seaweed
White peaches	Savoy cabbage	Soybeans	Walnuts	Wheat bran

Lots of the recipes which are included in Part 3 are rich in prebiotic and probiotic foods.

What About Alcohol?

Lots of people ask when they can reintroduce alcohol. You can reintroduce it in Stage 2 in moderation, but I would recommend that if you do wish to reintroduce alcohol, opt for red wine (keeping to the government-recommended limit of 14 units per week) with your evening meal. Red wine is packed with a health-promoting polyphenol called resveratrol, which exerts numerous benefits on health, such as reducing the risk of heart disease, decreasing inflammation and boosting cognitive function. Polyphenols have been demonstrated to exert beneficial prebiotic effects, which can help promote gut health. In addition, red wine can boost the number of beneficial gut bacteria while decreasing harmful bacteria.

However, research has shown that alcohol – particularly in large amounts – and its metabolites can lead to gut inflammation and overwhelm the gastrointestinal tract and liver, resulting in damage to the gut as well as other organs.[3]

Avoidance of Additives

Research has suggested that permanent exposure of human gut microbiota to even low levels of additives may change the composition and function of gut microbiota, therefore impacting the immune system. This could potentially, at least in part, explain the increasing incidence of allergies and autoimmune diseases.

The effect of food additives on our gut bacteria has long been overlooked, but recently, several studies have determined that some gut microbiota are highly sensitive to preservatives. One study found that the bacteria they tested exhibited a wide range of susceptibilities to food additives – for example, the most susceptible strain, *Bacteroides coprocola*, was almost 580 times more susceptible to sodium nitrite than the most resistant strain, *Enterococcus faecalis*.[4] Most significantly, the researchers found that gut microbes with known anti-inflammatory properties, such as *Clostridium tyrobutyricum* or *Lactobacillus paracasei*, were significantly more susceptible to additives than microbes with known pro-inflammatory properties, such as *Bacteroides thetaiotaomicron* or *Enterococcus faecalis*.

Other categories of additives have also been demonstrated to exert negative effects on human health. This includes dietary emulsifiers, which can directly change the composition of the human gut microbiota and trigger intestinal inflammation.[5] Therefore, during your time following the Good Gut Health Plan and once you have finished the programme, I would highly recommend you limit your intake of chemical additives, and this includes additives that sneak their way into supplements, which we will explore in Chapter 11.

Summary

Gut health has a huge impact on our immunity and also plays an essential role in autoimmune healing and reducing our risk of allergies. To balance and heal the immune system, we need to repair the gut lining and concentrate on strengthening the gut barrier to decrease our risk of experiencing leaky gut. This is very important as it will help to improve the immune response. A compromised gut barrier can allow undigested food particles and other substances to enter the bloodstream, triggering an inappropriate immune response and inflammation. So, if you are experiencing dysbiosis and/or leaky gut syndrome, focusing on treating these two gut issues is crucial. A balanced and diverse gut microbiome is vital for the proper development and regulation of the immune system.

CHAPTER 7

How to Eat for a Balanced Immune System – Macronutrients

Food and nutrition are our most accessible and powerful tools when it comes to improving our immune health and reducing inflammation, and diversity in our diet is vital for optimal immunity. But we are all unique in our genes, tastes, backgrounds, experiences and lifestyles, which means that our approaches to diet, nutrition and food are going to be different.

The aim here is to cultivate a diet that is nutritious, varied and nourishing and which works for you as an individual. In this chapter we are going to explore how our nutrition, diet and food choices can be improved, and how through these powerful tools at our fingertips we can actually reduce our risk of allergies, autoimmune disease and infectious disease, and optimize immune function.

Food is a medicine providing us with:

- essential nutrients that are involved in hundreds of chemical reactions in our body
- the required energy we need so we can launch an immune response
- building blocks to make new cells
- vital resources to make antibodies
- antioxidants that help protect our cells

HOW TO EAT FOR A BALANCED IMMUNE SYSTEM – MACRONUTRIENTS

- anti-inflammatory properties to combat harmful inflammation.

Calories are a currency of energy, and our immune system relies on sufficient calorie intake to carry out its many roles. Without adequate calorie intake, immunity can be compromised and impaired, and we will lack what we need to launch an effective immune response. However, it is all about balance, and too many calories can be as detrimental as too few calories. If you are consuming too many calories, this can lead to overnutrition and an inflammatory status which may impact your immune health significantly. What we eat can impact our immunity massively, so focusing on how we can improve and support our immune health through the food we eat is our ultimate goal.

So – what exactly should we be eating then, and how much? Well, the role of the macronutrients (carbohydrates, protein and fat) is crucial when it comes to immune health, so let's look at these three major food groups first.

Carbohydrates

Carbohydrates, often referred to as carbs, have had a bad press over the last decade or so, but they are essential for health. In fact, carbohydrates are the main source of fuel for the immune system and the brain. When we are fighting an infection, our immune cells' preferred fuel source is glucose, and if we don't have adequate glucose, this can affect our immune system's ability to fight infection. It may also result in a decreased number of essential immune cells as well as impact their function.[1]

However, not all carbohydrate foods are created equal or provide the same benefits to our health. To obtain the beneficial effects that carbs provide, we need to focus on including in our diet the most nutritious carbohydrate sources available, which are known as complex carbohydrates. Foods rich in complex carbs include wholegrain foods, such as rye bread, brown rice and whole-grain pasta. At the same time we should aim to limit or avoid foods high in simple carbohydrates, which are refined grain foods, such as white bread, white pasta and cereals. These are simple carbohydrate foods that have been processed to remove the outer bran and germ layers of the grain, leaving only the starchy endosperm. These grains are processed to increase shelf life, which can also make them more affordable. In addition to removing the fibre of the food, though, this processing removes key essential nutrients, such as some of the B vitamins and minerals like iron. Sometimes the food manufacturers will 'fortify' the food by adding the removed nutrients back in.

> Studies have shown that **high-carb meals** can result in higher oxidative stress and inflammation.

Complex carbohydrates consist of sugar molecules that are linked together in long chains and are found in foods such as chickpeas, beans and different vegetables. These foods take longer to digest, and as they are packed with fibre, this can help prevent blood-sugar spikes.

Simple carbohydrates, on the other hand, consist of single sugar molecules, known as monosaccharides, or two sugar molecules bonded together, known as disaccharides. Simple carbs can be found naturally in foods such as fruit but also as added sugars in other foods, including cakes, biscuits and sweets. These foods are quickly digested and absorbed, and subsequently, they provide a quick boost of energy that causes a quick rise in blood-sugar levels. Foods rich in simple carbohydrates tend to contain fewer vitamins, minerals and fibre than complex carbohydrate foods.

> **Simple carbohydrates** include monosaccharides (glucose, fructose and galactose) and disaccharides (sucrose – i.e. table sugar – lactose and maltose). They are found in foods such as fruit, milk, honey, syrup, sweets, sugar-sweetened soft drinks, baked goods and many other processed foods.

The key is to know how to choose carbohydrates so you are getting the most nutrition possible from your food with the least impact on your blood sugar, as balanced blood sugar is vital for immune health. If blood-sugar levels remain elevated for too long, this can impact our immune cells' ability to function, increasing our risk of infections. For optimal immunity we should prioritize complex, fibre-rich carbohydrates that are rich in vitamins, minerals, phytonutrients (powerful plant chemicals) and antioxidants. These complex carbohydrates that are high in fibre will take longer to digest, meaning they have a less immediate impact on our blood sugar, so it increases more slowly.

Fibre

Fibre is a carbohydrate found in plants. There are different types of fibre, such as soluble, which can dissolve in water, and insoluble fibre. Most plant foods contain both soluble and insoluble fibre; however, some foods are richer in one type of fibre than the other.

Soluble fibre can switch immune cells from a pro-inflammatory status to anti-inflammatory, allowing us to recover more quickly from an infection.[2] In addition, soluble fibre can 'feed' our beneficial gut bacteria, helping them to thrive. Insoluble fibre is different, as it is not fermented in the colon and doesn't 'feed' our beneficial bacteria. It is, however, key for aiding regular and healthy bowel movement.

A certain form of soluble fibre is known as prebiotic fibre, and this type of fibre serves as a primary food source for our beneficial gut bacteria and supports their growth and activity. These bacteria, in turn, then produce beneficial substances like short-chain fatty acids (SCFAs) that benefit our health. Prebiotic fibre provides vital fuel for our gut microbes, and if we don't include adequate amounts in our diet, this can have a negative impact on our immune health and may lead to illness.[3] By fuelling our gut bacteria with the most appropriate nutrition for them, we are also ensuring optimal immune health.

Two types of soluble fibre that promote the growth of our beneficial microbes are beta-glucan and inulin. Beta-glucan, which is present in oats and barley, has been confirmed to improve immune response and have antimicrobial and anti-inflammatory properties.[4] Meanwhile, inulin can be found in onions, leeks, garlic and a type of artichoke known as Jerusalem artichoke – in fact, the inulin in Jerusalem artichoke makes up 70 per cent of the fibre in the vegetable. However, while inulin can be very beneficial to health, it can cause symptoms such as bloating and gas in some people who struggle to tolerate high FODMAP foods. Therefore, it is sensible when increasing your intake of inulin foods to start with eating smaller servings to prevent any uncomfortable side effects. Increasing intake slowly will allow your body the time to adjust to the fibre in these healthful foods.

> **FODMAP** refers to fermentable oligosaccharides, disaccharides, monosaccharides and polyols, which are carbohydrates that are poorly absorbed in the small intestine and can cause digestive issues in some individuals.

There is also a third type of fibre, known as resistant starch because it is not able to be digested anywhere apart from the colon. Resistant starch helps support both immune and gut health, and once it reaches the colon our gut microbes 'feed' on it and produce an SCFA called butyrate. This is the beneficial SCFA which helps to reduce inflammation as well as supports our important gut barrier, helping to keep potentially harmful pathogens out.

Good sources of resistant starch are cooled down potatoes, green (unripe) bananas and legumes.

Since different types of fibre are found in different proportions in fibre-containing foods and have different properties, it is essential that we include lots of diversity in our diet and focus on eating different fibre-containing foods.

THE BENEFITS OF FIBRE

Fibre is such an important nutrient as it promotes health in numerous ways:

- supports digestive health
- prevents constipation
- reduces the risk of heart disease and stroke
- decreases the risk of type 2 diabetes
- improves blood pressure levels
- improves cholesterol levels

- reduces bowel cancer risk
- provides the 'fuel' for our gut bacteria to carry out their important functions.

A significant benefit of fibre is the role it plays in weight management and metabolic health as it can help you feel fuller for longer and it slows the digestion of food. Fibre reduces the glycaemic index of food, which is how quickly you absorb the sugars. If you remove fibre from a food, then you are absorbing the glucose from it quickly, which can lead to feeling hungry sooner than if you had eaten a food with its fibre intact. If you are fuller for longer, this means you are less likely to snack and will go for longer between meals.

The human diet has been subject to huge changes over the last few hundred years, and this is a vital consideration in explaining the significant difference in the prevalence of chronic metabolic disease between developed and developing nations. Unfortunately, the gap created by decreased fibre intake has now been filled by the increased intake of energy-dense, high-glycaemic load foods that make up a massive part of the average Western diet.

> Only 4 per cent of women and 13 per cent of men consume the recommended **30g** of fibre a day.

Studies have confirmed that individuals from industrialized Western nations consume approximately 12–18g of fibre a day,[5] compared with those from non-industrialized nations, who are eating up to 50g a day.[6] Current recommendations for fibre intake are 25–32g per day for women and 30–35g per day for men.[7] However, populations in the Western world are still way off meeting these guidelines.

> Our ancestors are believed to have eaten a whopping **100g of fibre** a day.[8]

Many people who are fibre-deficient are consuming ultra-processed diets that are high in added sugar as well as saturated and trans fats, which are having a significant impact on their immunity, gut health and overall health. One study demonstrated the importance of switching to a high-fibre diet by concluding that for every 1,000 people who changed from a low-fibre diet (less than 15g) to a high-fibre diet (25-29g), thirteen deaths and six cases of heart disease would be prevented.[9]

There is substantial evidence that diet–microbiome interactions are critical in the ability of fibre to improve chronic gut diseases as well as metabolic health in individuals who are obese and have metabolic syndrome.[10] Although further research is needed regarding dietary fibre and microbiome interactions, based on the current evidence that we have, it does appear to be a promising and cost-effective method to help decrease metabolic disease.

Additionally, a healthy gastrointestinal tract is essential for healthy, balanced immunity because if we are constantly constipated, it can result in toxin build-up that could be absorbed into the bloodstream, leading to some very nasty symptoms. Ultimately, without a sufficient intake of fibre, our immune function will be adversely impacted and compromised. Focus on including a wide variety of different whole grains, fruits, vegetables, legumes, nuts and seeds in your daily diet. These foods are rich in complex carbs that support our gut health, which in turn further supports our immune health.

HOW MUCH FIBRE IS IN THE FOOD WE EAT?

Fibre exists in food in very different amounts. Here is the fibre content of some of the most common foods many of us eat:

- 100g whole-grain pasta – 12g
- 200g tinned baked beans – 10g
- 1 medium baked potato (180g) – 5g
- 50g oats – 4g
- 2 slices whole-grain bread – 4g
- 80g cooked chickpeas – 4g
- 80g cooked lentils – 3g
- 100g dried brown rice – 2g
- handful of nuts – 2g
- 1 medium banana – 2g

What you would need to eat to reach the daily 30g recommended amount:

- 50g oats – **4g**
- 2 thick slices whole-grain toast – **4g**
- 200g tinned baked beans – **10g**
- 1 medium baked potato (180g) – **5g**
- 1 cup of broccoli – **5g**
- 1 apple – **2g**

It is fairly easy to reach the recommended 30g a day once you know the fibre content of the foods you eat.

HOW TO EAT FOR A BALANCED IMMUNE SYSTEM – MACRONUTRIENTS

TOP TIPS

- When it comes to fruits and vegetables, eat the edible peel, if possible, as this is a simple and easy way to boost your intake of fibre.
- Replace white carbohydrate foods with the whole-grain varieties.
- Bulk out meals such as curries, casseroles and soups with extra vegetables, lentils or beans.
- If you eat snacks, instead of reaching for the biscuit tin, eat oatcakes, nuts or vegetable sticks, such as red pepper, celery or cucumber, and dip into hummus.

Important – if you don't currently eat much fibre, increase the amount you eat slowly to avoid any digestive issues.

Phytonutrients

Phytonutrients, also known as phytochemicals, are also found in abundance in plant foods, and these very important nutrients have also been shown to have a significant impact on gut and immune health. Phytonutrients are compounds that are made by plants, and numerous studies have confirmed that they can decrease inflammation and combat free radicals, thereby preventing damage to our cells which could lead to potential illness and disease.

> Factors that can cause your body to produce **excessive free radicals** include consuming a low-nutrient diet, drinking alcohol and smoking tobacco. Eating a diet rich in antioxidants can help your body counter oxidative stress caused by excess free radicals and other toxins that increase your risk of disease.

It is estimated that there are over 25,000 different phytonutrients from different phytochemical classes which exert different benefits on our health. Research has shown that fruits, vegetables and grains contain more than 5,000 different types of phytonutrients, and some wholefoods may contain up to a whopping 25,000 individual phytonutrients.[11] This is why it is so important to consume the best carbohydrate sources we can, as then we can reap the health benefits these foods and nutrients provide. Let's take a look at some of the most common phytonutrients.

POLYPHENOLS

When it comes to phytonutrients, one of the most studied classes are polyphenols, which are a large and diverse family of plant compounds characterized as having two or more phenol groups in their structure. Polyphenols are among the most abundant chemicals in the plant kingdom, interacting with the intestinal immune system, which may lead to potentially beneficial effects on health.[12]

Polyphenols support health in numerous ways, such as:

- supporting immune function
- reducing cancer risk
- enhancing antitumour immunity
- promoting immunity to harmful pathogens

- regulating intestinal mucosal immune responses
- reducing our risk of allergic disease
- promoting gut health.

Decades of research analysing polyphenols have resulted in numerous insights regarding the impact of polyphenols on immune function. Current research strongly suggests that polyphenols can help to prevent several immune diseases.[13]

They are found in many plant foods, particularly fruits and vegetables, and many high-quality studies have confirmed that consumption of these plant compounds can decrease the incidence of chronic diseases. Consuming plant foods in our daily diets is the most bioavailable approach to benefit from these beneficial phytochemicals.

> **Polyphenols** can regulate the immune response as well as inflammation by acting as anti-inflammatory and antioxidant agents.

Polyphenols can play an essential role in our gut microbial community as they exert positive effects on our beneficial gut microbes. These powerful plant compounds may modify immune function by changing our gut microbiota. We know how closely immune and gut health are; therefore, by improving our gut health, this in turn will support our immune health.

This category of phytonutrients includes flavonoids, which have impressive anti-inflammatory, antimicrobial and antioxidant properties. This phytonutrient can be found in foods such as apples, coffee, ginger, onions and cacao (dark chocolate with minimum 70 per cent cacao). Flavonoids can combat harmful free radicals that can harm and damage our cells and they also play an important and effective role in reducing our risk of infections and chronic disease.

> **Did you know?** Vitamin P was the term once used for the group of plant compounds called flavonoids, which are found in citrus fruits, berries, different vegetables and tea.

CAROTENOIDS

Carotenoids, like polyphenols, have anti-inflammatory and antioxidant properties.[14] There are hundreds of different carotenoids, including beta-carotene, lutein, lycopene and zeaxanthin, and they can be found in foods such as kale, spinach, carrots, sweet potatoes and cantaloupe melon.

> **Carotenoids** are **fat-soluble** so it is advisable to eat a carotenoid food with a fat source, such as cheese or olive oil, as this will promote optimal nutrient absorption.

Carotenoids are sometimes described as polyphenols, although they are structurally different. However, both are responsible for the vibrant colours in plants, have antioxidant and anti-inflammatory properties and provide health-promoting effects.

To ensure you are getting a wide variety of different phytonutrients in your daily diet, focus on including lots of different plant foods and don't consume the same fruits, vegetables, herbs, spices or grains – aim to mix things up. By doing this you will get the maximum health benefits that these wonderful plant chemicals provide.

HOW TO EAT FOR A BALANCED IMMUNE SYSTEM – MACRONUTRIENTS

Myconutrients

A myconutrient is the fungi and yeast form of a plant phytonutrient and is just as powerful as its plant equivalent, with its anti-inflammatory, antioxidant and antiviral properties helping to support normal functioning of our immune system. The immune-supporting activity of mushrooms is due to the unique nutrients present, and different mushrooms possess their own myconutrients. These magical myconutrients in functional mushrooms also act as biological response modifiers, meaning that they can support different arms of the immune response as well as protect against infection, inflammatory diseases and allergies.

> **Medicinal mushrooms** are often known as functional mushrooms and have specific medicinal properties, differentiating them from their culinary counterparts.

The most well-studied myconutrient in mushrooms is beta-D-glucans (or beta-glucans), a nourishing nutrient that influences our immune health significantly. Several immune cells possess receptors which recognize beta-glucans and result in an increased resistance to infection and potentially cancer.[15] Beta-glucans also act as a prebiotic fibre and 'feed' our beneficial gut bacteria. Other myconutrients can be found in functional mushrooms but these tend to be specific to the individual mushroom and have their own special properties and benefits.

Numerous types of medicinal mushrooms help to support the immune system. The mushroom cordyceps has been reported to reduce bacterial load in the lungs, promote immune response and reduce inflammation. A 2019 study confirmed that supplementing with 1.7g of cordyceps mycelium culture extract resulted in a 38 per cent increase in the activity of natural killer cells, which help protect against infection. In addition, powerful phenolic acids in mushrooms such as the reishi and chaga modulate the immune response, preventing inflammation by acting on enzymes like cyclooxygenase-2 (COX-2) that are the target of certain medications including aspirin and ibuprofen. These powerful compounds, along with other bioactive compounds, are also thought to play a role in the mushrooms' anti-inflammatory, anticancer and antioxidant properties.

> **Ergosterol** is a plant-based precursor of vitamin D2. When mushrooms are exposed to sunlight they convert this to vitamin D2, an essential immune-nourishing nutrient.

Protein

Proteins are known as the building blocks of life and are basically large molecules made up of lots of small molecules, known as amino acids, which are linked together in long chains. How the amino acids are ordered determines the structure and function of each individual protein.

There are 20 types of amino acids that combine to make a protein. We can make eleven of these amino acids ourselves, and these are known as 'non-essential amino acids', while the remaining nine amino acids, referred to as 'essential amino acids', we can't make ourselves, so we need to obtain these through our diet. Obtaining the correct balance of these amino acids is very important for immune health as they are involved in making immune cells as well as antibodies to combat infection.

You may have heard the term 'complete protein', which refers to a food that contains all nine essential amino acids. Excellent complete protein sources include meat, fish, eggs, dairy and certain plant sources, such as soy products (tofu, edamame beans) and the grain quinoa. Animal food sources have in the past been considered the ideal complete protein foods as they have a higher content of the amino acid leucine. However, leucine is also found in plant foods such as soy products (tofu, edamame and tempeh), lentils, beans, chickpeas, nuts, seeds and mushrooms. If you follow a vegan eating plan, then focus on including lots of these different plant-based leucine food sources to ensure you meet the recommended requirement of this amino acid.

We also have incomplete protein foods, which contain some of the essential amino acids but not all. Many plant-based protein food sources, such as nuts, seeds and most grains, are considered incomplete proteins and need to be eaten along with another incomplete protein, either in a meal or at different points of the day. So, for example, you may have beans or lentils in one meal and rice in another. I find it easier to include them at the same time together – for example, rice and beans in a chilli – as this will help to promote the usability of protein. These two foods when eaten together will provide all nine essential amino acids, thereby making them a complete protein source. Focus on including a variety of plant protein every day and this will ensure you are getting all the essential amino acids you need.

There is growing evidence that swapping a diet that is focused on animal protein, such as chicken, meat and fish, for a diet that is high in plant protein, such as grains, nuts and pulses, could help us live longer. In 2016, new guidelines were introduced, placing greater emphasis on including non-meat sources of protein in our diets.[16] So, we don't need to give up meat, eggs and dairy products entirely, but instead include more plant food sources in our diet.

This will have the added benefit of providing lots of fibre and phytonutrients while being much more cost-effective, too, so it's a win-win situation!

> Our **gut microbes** can make small amounts of **protein** – another way they help us!

Proteins have several important roles, such as aiding growth, repair, function and structure for our tissues and organs. This essential macronutrient is also vital for strong and balanced immunity. Protein also provides the building blocks that support immunity by making new immune cells and antibodies, and it also allows the immune system to mount an immune response when needed. Several studies have confirmed that protein deficiency can harm immune function as well as increase the risk of infectious disease.[17] Also, if there is too little protein in your diet, you may experience symptoms such as low energy, tiredness and weakness. We need to ensure we eat enough protein to stave off these unwanted symptoms.

> All the **cells** in our body contain protein!

So, exactly how much protein should we be eating? Well, there has been a lot of conversation recently around the amount of protein we should be consuming, but current UK guidelines suggest that adult women should aim for approximately 45g per day while men should consume 56g per day. This is equivalent to approximately two portions of meat, poultry, fish, tofu or nuts a day – as a very

HOW TO EAT FOR A BALANCED IMMUNE SYSTEM – MACRONUTRIENTS

rough guide, a serving of protein should fit into the palm of your hand. US guidelines are similar and suggest 0.8g of protein per kg of body weight, which is approximately 46g for the average sedentary woman and 56g for the average sedentary man.

In times of illness or recuperating from surgery, it is advisable to include foods that are rich in the amino acids arginine and glutamine. These two amino acids are non-essential amino acids, but during an immune response they actually become conditionally essential, as when we are ill, they are used at an increased rate by the immune system, helping prevent inflammatory responses when recuperating from illness. Foods that are rich in these amino acids include chicken as well as plant sources such as legumes, beans and nuts.

> **Arginine** is important for immune function, collagen production and wound healing. During times of stress like illness or surgery, arginine can be depleted, making it even more important to ensure adequate intake.
>
> **Glutamine** helps protect cells during stress, such as at time of illness or injury, and is also important for immune function, collagen production and wound healing.

If you are experiencing significant stress, then you may need to up your protein intake. Additionally, for individuals over the age of 65, it may be sensible to eat more than the recommended amount, as doing so will limit age-associated muscle loss.[18] An ideal amount for older individuals would be between 1–1.2g per kg of body weight, so for a 64kg individual, this would be between 64–77g of protein a day.

A lot of people think that they don't eat enough protein, but in the UK, many of us are actually eating more protein than is recommended as per the official dietary guidelines. This is not necessarily an issue, but it depends on the protein that you are consuming, as diets that are heavy in meat have been associated with an increased risk of type 2 diabetes, heart disease and some cancers. However, meat is a significant source of vitamin B12, so if you plan to reduce your meat consumption, it is important to make sure you are including other sources of vitamin B12, such as fish, eggs or fortified foods, including nutritional yeast, breakfast cereals and some plant-based milks. Try to include one protein serving, around the size of your palm, in each meal of the day.

Also, it is important to eat no more than 70g of red and processed cooked meat a day, as per NHS recommendations. Processed meat is any meat that has been preserved by curing, smoking, salting or adding preservatives, and includes sausages, bacon, ham, salami, corned beef and pâtés.

As you can see from the table below, it is very easy to exceed the recommended 70g of red and processed meat. If you do exceed this amount one day, then the next day eat less or no red meat so that you average out at no more than 70g a day over the course of a week.

Average weight of red and processed meat servings:

- 1 slice of ham – 23g
- 1 slice of corned beef – 38g
- Quarter-pound beef burger – 78g (cooked weight)
- 140g (5oz) rump steak – 102g (cooked weight)
- 2 sausages and 2 thin bacon rashers – 130g
- 225g (8oz) beef steak – 163g (cooked weight)

HOW TO EAT FOR A BALANCED IMMUNE SYSTEM – MACRONUTRIENTS

Studies have linked high intakes of red and processed meat to an increased risk of bowel cancer. Processed meat can also be high in salt, which can increase your blood sugar, and high in saturated fat, which may increase blood cholesterol levels if you consume too much of it. Having high cholesterol can increase your risk of coronary heart disease. Instead of eating processed meat, aim to eat more beans, chickpeas, lentils, peas, nuts and seeds and ideally two servings of fish a week, one serving being an oily fish such as salmon, sardines, trout or mackerel.

It is also important to note that mock vegetarian or vegan meat alternatives contain protein, but they can be packed with salt, sugar and saturated fat. Therefore, to obtain the full benefits that plant protein provides, aim to replace meat with more pulses, whole grains and soy, such as tofu and miso.

> **An average adult woman** would need to eat approximately one serving each of meat and tofu a day, or one serving each of fish and chicken a day, to meet the UK and US daily recommended amount of protein. However, the amount needed to meet daily recommendations varies based on individual factors like body weight and activity level.

Fats

Like carbohydrates, dietary fats have had a bad press in the past. However, this macronutrient is vital for immunity and many other areas of health:

- acting as building blocks for cells
- producing hormones

- reducing inflammation
- providing energy
- absorbing the fat-soluble vitamins A, D, E and K
- helping to regulate blood sugar.

As with protein and carbohydrates, there are different types of fat and some are associated with beneficial effects on health, whereas others are more harmful.

Diets that are high in fat can change our gut bacteria and are also associated with a reduction in bacteria diversity. In addition, eating a high-fat diet can result in too high an energy intake, leading to potential weight gain and body fat accumulation.

Foods tend to have a combination of the different types of fat, and some are essential, whereas others are not. We want to focus on including the essential fats, known as EFAs.

The 'Healthy' Fats

Polyunsaturated fats are also known as PUFAs, and as our body is unable to make these fats, we need to obtain them from the food we eat. This type of fat can be found in oils such as sunflower oil and safflower oil. PUFAs are important as they are involved in our cell membrane structure, play a vital role in regulating blood pressure, reduce inflammation and support our nervous system. They have also been shown, when unheated, to decrease heart disease risk and support our immune system.

Two types of polyunsaturated fats are omega-3 and omega-6 fatty acids; these are known as essential fats, which we need to get from our diets. They are vital fats as they play a critical role in immune cell function, digestion, brain function, blood clotting and the movement of cholesterol within the body. They have also been shown to be protective and can help decrease inflammation, with researchers consistently confirming the association between an increased omega-3 intake and decreased inflammation.

Omega-3 fatty acids can also help to treat autoimmune conditions, such as rheumatoid arthritis, Crohn's disease, psoriasis, ulcerative colitis and lupus. Consuming an adequate omega-3 intake in the first 12 months of life is associated with a reduced risk of autoimmunity.

The three main omega-3 fatty acids are EPA, DHA and ALA. Animal products, including fatty fish, such as salmon, mackerel and trout, are excellent sources of EPA and DHA, while you can find ALA in plant-based foods such as walnuts, chia seeds and flaxseeds (linseeds).

Omega-6 fatty acids are also considered essential, and like omega-3 they need to be obtained through the food we eat. These fats are found in lots of different foods, such as sunflower oil, safflower oil, walnuts, cashews, almonds, farmed fish and many ultra-processed foods. When it comes to omega-3 and omega-6, we want to make sure that they are balanced, as recent research has indicated that the omega-6 and omega-3 ratio is critical to preventing the development of metabolic disorders that may increase cardiovascular disease risk. The human body can maintain optimum health with an intake ratio of omega-6:omega-3 of 5:1; however, the current ratio is 20:1 in the Western diet.[19] As the consumption of a heavy omega-6 PUFA diet increases, researchers have observed an increase in the incidence rate of metabolic syndromes through activating the inflammatory pathways. Omega-6 and omega-3 compete for the same enzyme binding site, and depending on which is bound, the resulting essential fatty acid signals a cascade of pro-inflammatory or anti-inflammatory factors.[20]

> **Omega-3 fatty acids** promote anti-inflammatory responses, while an excessive omega-6 intake can result in a cascade of circulating pro-inflammatory factors.

Researchers have suggested that the best approach to lower the average of 20:1 omega-6:omega-3 ratio is to start by decreasing omega-6 intake while increasing omega-3 intake. Including foods such as seafood, nuts and seeds may be helpful, as these foods have been the focus of studies that have confirmed the positive and beneficial effects of omega-3 fatty acids in the diet.[21] There are no current official recommendations as to how much omega-3 we should be consuming in our diets; however, it is generally acknowledged that two servings of fish a week is acceptable, one being an oily fish, such as salmon, sardines or trout. If you cannot eat fish, then you may wish to consider algae supplements as an alternative.

Another type of 'healthy' fat is monounsaturated fat (MUFA). This type of fatty acid is found in abundance in foods such as olive oil, avocado, nuts and seeds. MUFAs provide beneficial effects on health, such as reducing inflammation, promoting optimal immune function and potentially enhancing our immune system's ability to fight off infections and diseases.

The 'Not So Healthy' Fats

While monounsaturated and polyunsaturated fats have been shown to decrease inflammation, researchers have confirmed that saturated fat can promote an inflammatory response. This type of fat is solid at room temperature and is found in animal products such as fatty meats, cheese, butter, lard and ghee. Numerous studies have highlighted that swapping saturated fat with healthier fat may reduce heart disease.

Easy ways to cut down on saturated fat are to opt for lower-fat meats, such as chicken and turkey, remove all skin and fat from the meat, and choose healthy monounsaturated fat sources to cook with, such as olive oil instead of butter, which is high in saturated fat. Saturated fat products can still be included in the diet, but it is important to keep to the daily recommended intake, which for women is no more than 20g and for men 30g or less.[22]

The nutrition labels on food packaging can also help you cut down on total fat and saturated fat. However, be aware that foods that are lower in fat are not necessarily lower in calories, and sometimes the fat is replaced with sugar and the food may end up having a similar energy content to the regular version. Becoming label-savvy is key!

> **High** in saturated fat – more than 5g of saturates per 100g.
> **Low** in saturated fat – 1.5g of saturates or less per 100g or 0.75g per 100ml for liquids.
> **Saturated fat-free** – 0.1g of saturates per 100g or 100ml.

Another fat that has been shown to promote inflammation is known as a trans fat, and this is a fat we want to avoid completely, if possible. These are polyunsaturated fats that, when they are heated, can become damaged and change into trans fats. These harmful fats have been confirmed to impact our immune health as well as fertility in women. Foods that contain trans fats are sweet, processed foods, such as cookies, pastries, ice cream and margarines that contain hydrogenated vegetable oils.

Trans fats exert many negative effects on health, so why are so many companies still using them? The answer most likely lies in the fact that trans fats are easy to use, inexpensive to produce and last a long time. They can also create a desirable taste and texture. Unlike saturated fats, which we have recommended intake guidelines to adhere to, there is no recommended or safe level for trans fats consumption. However, bans on trans fats currently exist in Canada, Denmark, Switzerland, Austria and certain US states, including New York and California. Disappointingly, a UK ban has not been met with government support; instead, food companies are allowed to reduce the trans fat content of their foods on a voluntary basis.[23] While many food manufacturers have decreased the amounts of these fats in their products, these harmful fats are still present in many foods. So, it is very important to read labels to see if any trans fats have sneaked their way into the food – look for the term 'mono and diglycerides of fatty acids' as this is a trans fat.

Summary

What we choose to eat is vital for immune health and reducing inflammation, and variety when it comes to diet is key to ensuring healthy immunity. A diet that is nutritious, diverse and balanced, and which works for you, is the ultimate goal. This will reduce your risk of allergy, autoimmune disease and infectious disease as well as optimize immune function. Focus on including a variety of whole-grain carbohydrates, high-quality protein foods and healthy fats to ensure your immune system is the healthiest and most balanced it can be.

CHAPTER 8

How to Eat for a Balanced Immune System – Micronutrients

The Micronutrients

Numerous different micronutrients are required to promote optimal immunity, and the best way to meet the daily requirements of these essential vitamins and minerals is to focus on eating a diverse and nutrient-dense diet. Even a slight deficiency in one of these important vitamins and minerals may have a significant effect on immune function as well as overall health.

Let's take a closer look at the vitamins that have been shown to support the health of our immune system.

The Water-Soluble Vitamins

VITAMIN C

Also known as ascorbic acid, vitamin C has powerful antioxidant, antimicrobial and anti-inflammatory properties and is widely used in the treatment of a variety of diseases.[1] It is an essential nutrient for a diverse range of immune functions, with research reporting that it may also provide beneficial effects against various viral infections.[2] Studies have also determined that if patients with pneumonia have intravenous vitamin C administered, they may experience less severe symptoms.[3]

In addition, there has been a huge amount of interest in vitamin C for the common cold since the middle of the 20th century. This powerful antioxidant vitamin has been confirmed to reduce the severity of common cold symptoms as well as the actual duration of the cold. One study found that regular vitamin C supplementation of at least 0.2 g/day shortened the duration of colds by 9.4 per cent.[4] However, while the available evidence shows that vitamin C can influence colds, the optimal dosage and the effect of the maximum benefit is not fully known at present.

Researchers have also been investigating the role of vitamin C in treating Covid-19 and found that it can reduce inflammation, improve oxygen support status and reduce mortality in Covid-19 patients, all without causing any negative side effects.[5]

> **Iron-deficient?** Then you may benefit from increasing your vitamin C intake, as vitamin C increases iron absorption.

When we are fighting an infection, our immune system uses up a lot more vitamin C, so we need to ensure we are eating lots of foods that are high in vitamin C, such as raspberries, strawberries, blueberries, oranges and kiwi fruit. If you don't feel up to eating, it may be helpful to include these fruits in a smoothie.

In addition to the significant benefits that vitamin C provides for immune health, as a potent antioxidant, it also promotes wound healing and supports the health of our bones, cartilage, blood vessels and skin. This essential micronutrient is also crucial for many metabolic reactions and antioxidant protection during exercise, as well as beneficial in promoting sleep duration, reducing sleep disturbances, relieving movement disorders and decreasing the dangerous effects of sleep apnoea.[6]

Recommendations for vitamin C intake for UK adults aged 19 to 64 is 40mg per day, and you should be able to reach this level from your food intake as long as you are meeting the government guidelines recommendation of 'five-a-day', which includes eating five portions of different vegetables and fruits per day. I would suggest three of these servings should be vegetables and two should be fruits. This recommendation was based on epidemiological evidence indicating an association between the consumption of more than 400g a day of fruits and vegetables with a decreased risk of certain diet-related chronic diseases, such as heart disease, stroke and some cancers.

The NHS defines an adult portion of fruits and vegetables to be 80g.[7] For fruit, this equates to:

- a small- or medium-sized apple, pear or orange
- two smaller fruits like clementines, apricots or plums
- a handful of grapes (approximately ten), strawberries or cherries.

In terms of vegetables, 80g would look like:

- two broccoli spears
- three celery sticks
- one medium tomato or seven cherry tomatoes
- eight small cauliflower florets
- two heaped tablespoons of cooked spinach
- four heaped tablespoons of peas or sweetcorn.

It is important to note that unsweetened 100 per cent fruit juice, vegetable juice and smoothies can only ever count as a maximum of one portion of your five-a-day. So, your combined total of drinks from fruit juice, vegetable juice and smoothies shouldn't be more than 150ml a day, which is basically a small glass.

> **Potatoes** don't count towards your five-a-day as they are classified nutritionally as a 'starchy' food.

In the US, the recommended daily amount of vitamin C is significantly different to that of the UK. In fact, global recommendations for daily vitamin C intake vary by more than five-fold. In the US, women are recommended to consume 75mg a day (85mg for pregnant women, and 120mg if breastfeeding) while for men it is 90mg. The US guidelines also advise that if you are a smoker, you will require 35mg more vitamin C a day.

Numerous authorities recommend the minimum amount of vitamin C as per the UK recommendation; however, this may not be meeting the health requirements of various subpopulations – such as those who are pregnant or breastfeeding, those who are obese or those who smoke – who have increased needs compared with the general population. Smoking rates continue to increase in some countries, and research indicates that smokers may benefit from daily intakes of at least 200mg of vitamin C. Also, with obesity rates increasing globally, as well as obesity-related comorbidities such as metabolic syndrome, diabetes and cardiovascular disease, more research is needed regarding appropriate vitamin C recommendations for different individuals.

If you are poorly and don't feel up to eating or drinking, then you may wish to supplement, but aim to supplement with a maximum of 1g (1,000mg) a day to prevent any gut discomfort and stomach upset.

VITAMIN B

Vitamin B complex is a group of eight vitamins that includes vitamins B1, B2, B3, B5, B6, B7, B9 and B12, and they are essential for many different roles in our body, including supporting our immune system. While each B vitamin has its own specific role, they also work together synergistically to support overall immune function and overall health.

However, of particular importance when it comes to our immune health are vitamins B6, B9 and B12. These B vitamins are involved in the production of immune cells and the regulation of immune responses. They also help the body produce antibodies and maintain the overall balance of the immune system.

Let's take a closer look at these three B vitamins which play a vital role in supporting our immune system.

Vitamin B6 (pyridoxine)
This B vitamin is crucial for making red blood cells and helping produce white blood cells and T cells, which are vital for fighting off infections. Individuals with the autoimmune condition rheumatoid arthritis often have low vitamin B6 levels, which tend to decrease with increased disease severity. The suboptimal vitamin B6 concentrations found in those with rheumatoid arthritis are due to the inflammation caused by the condition, and, in turn, they increase the inflammation associated with the disease. Although vitamin B6 supplements can correct vitamin B6 levels in those with rheumatoid arthritis, they do not stop the production of inflammatory cytokines or reduce levels of inflammatory markers.

In the UK, the daily requirement of vitamin B6 for adults is 1.2mg for women and 1.4mg for men. The recommendation in the US is similar to that of the UK, and advises both adult men and women aged 19–50 to aim for 1.3mg of vitamin B6 a day. However, for older adults (aged 51 and above) the recommended amounts are higher at 1.5mg for women and 1.7mg for men.

When supplementing with vitamin B6, like with all micronutrient supplementation, it is important not to take too much. Taking

200mg or more a day of vitamin B6 can lead to a loss of feeling in the arms and legs known as peripheral neuropathy. This will usually improve once you stop taking the supplements. But in a few cases when people have taken large amounts of vitamin B6, particularly for more than a few months, the effect can be permanent. The NHS recommends not to take more than 10mg of vitamin B6 a day in supplements, unless advised to by a doctor.[8]

Vitamin B9 (folic acid/folate)
This vitamin works with vitamin B12 to create new red blood cells and is also important for the proper functioning of white blood cells, which are vital for immune responses. Folate is the naturally occurring form of vitamin B9, whereas folic acid is the synthetic form that is often found in supplements or fortified foods.

When it comes to vitamin B9, UK recommendations suggest that adults need 200mcg (micrograms) a day. Most people should be able to get the amount of folate they need by eating a varied and balanced diet. However, if you're pregnant, trying for a baby or may potentially get pregnant, the NHS recommends that you take a 400mcg folic acid supplement daily until you're 12 weeks pregnant. This is to help prevent neural tube defects, such as spina bifida, in your baby. Some women have an increased risk of having a pregnancy affected by a neural tube defect and may be advised to take a higher dose of 5mg of folic acid each day until they are 12 weeks pregnant. This is unlikely to cause harm as it's taken on a short-term basis; however, it is very important to speak with your doctor first before supplementing with this higher dose.

It is important to highlight that taking doses of vitamin B9 higher than 1mg can potentially mask the symptoms of vitamin B12 deficiency, which can eventually damage the nervous system if it's not spotted and treated. This is particularly a concern for older

HOW TO EAT FOR A BALANCED IMMUNE SYSTEM – MICRONUTRIENTS

people because it becomes more difficult to absorb vitamin B12 as you get older.

Vitamin B12 (cobalamin)
Vitamin B12 is essential for cell health, red blood cell production and supporting the immune system. A deficiency in vitamin B12 can weaken the immune system and make the body more susceptible to illness. Furthermore, the B vitamins, particularly B12, are essential for the gut bacteria's growth and function. They act as nutrients for the bacteria and influence their diversity and composition.

Vitamin B12 is involved in nucleotide and methionine biosynthesis, which are important for gut bacteria, and can also promote the growth of beneficial bacteria that produce short-chain fatty acids (SCFAs), which have powerful anti-inflammatory effects and help to maintain our gut barrier integrity.

> Since a large part of the immune system is in the gut, the **B vitamins**, especially vitamin B12, can help to support a healthy gut microbiome.

For vitamin B12, the recommended daily intake in the UK is 1.5mcg for adults aged 19–64. The US recommended daily amount for both adult men and women is higher than that of the UK at 2.4mcg a day.

Individuals who follow a vegan diet are at an increased risk of vitamin B12 deficiency and may wish to supplement. However, there's not enough evidence to show what the effects may be of taking high doses of vitamin B12 supplements each day. If you do take vitamin B12 supplements, it is important not to take too much as this could be harmful. However, the NHS states that taking 2mg or less a day of vitamin B12 in supplement form is unlikely to cause any harm.

Deficiency
One of the major causes of immune deficiency globally is chronic malnutrition. Malnutrition, encompassing both undernutrition and overnutrition, can significantly impact the immune system and impair immune cell development, function and responses. It can also affect our T cell production and function, cytokine production and the ability of immune cells to fight off potentially harmful invaders.

A significant percentage of the global population consumes less than the recommended daily allowance of vitamin B, which may increase the risk of a dysregulated immune system. Deficiency in vitamin B has also been associated with several neurological disorders, including depression, anxiety, dementia and Alzheimer's disease. There are complex interactions between the immune system and nervous system, and it is becoming clear that the immune system plays an important role in the development of mental health disorders, including cognitive decline, anxiety, mood changes and depression.[9] In the UK, both vitamin B12 deficiency and B9 deficiency are more common in older people, affecting around 1 in 10 people aged 75 or over and 1 in 20 people aged 65–74.[10]

Pernicious anaemia is an autoimmune condition that affects the stomach and is the most common cause of vitamin B12 deficiency in the UK as your body is unable to absorb it from the food you eat. Vitamin B12 is combined with a protein called intrinsic factor in the stomach, and this mix of vitamin B12 and intrinsic factor is then absorbed into the body in a part of the gut called the distal ileum. While the exact cause of pernicious anaemia is unknown, it is most common in women around 60 years of age as well as in people with a family history of the condition and those with another autoimmune condition, such as vitiligo or Addison's disease.

Additionally, vitamin B12 or B9 deficiency anaemia occurs when a lack of these vitamins causes the body to produce abnormally large red blood cells that cannot function properly. Red blood cells are incredibly important as they carry oxygen around our body using a substance called haemoglobin.

> **Anaemia** is the general term for having either fewer red blood cells than normal or having an abnormally low amount of haemoglobin in each red blood cell.

Although it's uncommon, vitamin B12 or B9 deficiency with or without anaemia can lead to complications, particularly if you have been deficient in vitamin B12 or B9 for some time. Potential complications can include:

- problems with the nervous system
- fertility issues
- heart conditions
- pregnancy complications and birth defects.

Adults with severe anaemia are also at risk of developing heart failure.

Some complications improve with appropriate treatment, but others, such as problems with the nervous system, can sometimes be permanent. Certain groups of people can develop a vitamin B12 deficiency as a result of not getting enough vitamin B12 from their diet. A diet that includes meat, fish and dairy products usually provides enough vitamin B12, but people who do not regularly eat these foods can become deficient. Therefore, those who follow a vegan diet and do not take vitamin B12 supplements or eat foods fortified with vitamin B12 are at risk of deficiency. Vitamin B12 deficiency can also be treated with injections, and this will most likely continue until your vitamin B12 levels have normalized.

Some stomach conditions or stomach operations can prevent the absorption of enough vitamin B12. For example, a gastrectomy, a surgical procedure in which part of your stomach is removed, increases your risk of developing a vitamin B12 deficiency. Some conditions that affect your intestines can also stop you absorbing the required amount of vitamin B12. An example of this can be seen in Crohn's disease, which is a long-term condition that causes inflammation of the lining of the digestive system. If you are an individual with Crohn's, your body may not be getting the vitamin B12 it needs.

As with vitamin B12 deficiency anaemia, folate (B9) deficiency anaemia can develop for several reasons. It can be caused by a lack of dietary folate, which is more common in individuals who eat an ultra-processed, nutrient-devoid diet, or who eat a very restrictive diet that is low in folate, and in individuals who abuse alcohol. Sometimes your body may be unable to absorb folate as effectively as it should. This is usually caused by an underlying condition affecting your digestive system, such as coeliac disease. Some types of medicines can also reduce the amount of folate in your body or make the folate harder to absorb. These include some anticonvulsants, which are medications that are used to treat epilepsy. However, your doctor or medical practitioner will be aware of medicines that can affect your folate levels and will monitor you if necessary. Premature babies, born before the 37th week of pregnancy, are also more likely to develop a folate deficiency because their developing bodies require higher amounts of folate than normal.

It is important to see your doctor or medical practitioner if you're experiencing symptoms of folate or B12 deficiency anaemia. These conditions can often be diagnosed based on your symptoms and the results of a blood test. It's important for vitamin B12 or folate deficiency anaemia to be diagnosed and treated as soon as possible, and although many of the symptoms improve with treatment, some issues can be potentially irreversible if not treated. Unfortunately, the longer the condition remains unaddressed, the greater the risk of long-term damage.

The Fat-Soluble Vitamins

VITAMIN D

Vitamin D plays a vital role in maintaining a healthy immune system. A deficiency in this micronutrient can weaken our immunity significantly and increase our susceptibility to infections. Sufficient vitamin D levels can strengthen immunity and help combat viral and bacterial infections effectively. Appropriate vitamin D intake may also help regulate immune responses to prevent excessive inflammation, which may lead to chronic disease.

Currently, vitamin D deficiency is a worldwide health concern and is believed to be mainly due to inadequate sunlight exposure. It is thought that approximately 1 billion individuals worldwide have vitamin D deficiency and almost 50 per cent of some populations have vitamin D insufficiency.

Increasing research has concluded that low vitamin D status is associated with a wide range of disorders, including autoimmune diseases such as multiple sclerosis, lupus and type 1 diabetes.

In addition, vitamin D is a key player between our immune system and gut microbiome, and low levels of vitamin D can impact the gut barrier, making it more permeable, thereby increasing our risk of leaky gut. Vitamin D deficiency can also adversely impact the balance of our gut microbiome, which can further affect immunity.

The good news is that the composition of our beneficial gut bacteria can be improved with optimal vitamin D levels, so ensuring we get the required amount of vitamin D is vital.

This essential nutrient is also involved in the activation of our immune cells, specifically the T cells, and it 'primes' them so they are prepared to respond more effectively to recognize, fight and destroy infectious and harmful pathogens. It can also support our other immune cells by promoting activity of our regulatory T cells (Tregs) that help to suppress inflammation, as well as supporting the development and function of our natural killer (NK) T cells, which play a vital role in immune responses.

In addition to immune support, vitamin D is vital for bone health as it regulates the amount of calcium and phosphate in the body. A vitamin D deficiency can result in a disease called rickets, which primarily affects infants and young children. In this condition, the growing bones fail to develop properly due to a lack of vitamin D, which results in soft and weakened bones, fractures, bone and muscle pain, and bone deformities. Rickets was common in the past, but it has mostly disappeared in the Western world, particularly after foods like margarine and cereal became fortified with the micronutrient. However, in recent years, there's been an increase in cases of rickets in the UK, and while the number of cases is still relatively small, research has confirmed that a significant number of individuals in the UK have low vitamin D levels in their blood. Children who do not have sufficient vitamin D or calcium, either through their diet or from sunlight, are at an increased risk of potentially developing rickets. The condition is more common in children with dark skin, as they need more sunlight to get enough vitamin D, as well as children born prematurely and those taking medication that interferes with vitamin D.[11]

> **Osteomalacia** is the adult form of a condition that is similar to rickets and with the same underlying issue of soft bones.

Official UK guidelines have advised that everyone should be supplementing with 10mcg of vitamin D from October through to April. In the US, a higher intake for all adults aged 19–70 is recommended at 15mcg. Again, these guidelines are at population level and are not a personalized recommendation for each and every one of us. I have seen a huge number of people who have followed this recommendation and subsequently been found to have dangerously high and toxic levels of vitamin D. This may be as some people only need vitamin D for one or two of the dark winter months, for example.

Vitamin D is mainly synthesized through exposing our skin to the sun's UV rays, and as we store vitamin D in our bodies, we can actually 'bank' vitamin D from the sunny summer months, which is something not a lot of people realize. However, research investigating vitamin D storage in adipose tissue (basically body fat) has been well established. Personally, I only supplement with vitamin D for two months in the year – February and March – as my vitamin D levels tend to be in the normal range from October to January. I would recommend, if possible, that you check your vitamin D levels with an at-home finger-prick test before you supplement with vitamin D to see if your current levels are normal or if they are low and you would benefit from supplementation – this could also save you money in the long term.

> Baring your face and arms for **10–15 minutes** several times a week is enough to keep vitamin D levels topped up for most people.

Sunlight is so important for producing vitamin D, and researchers have reported that through a separate mechanism to that of vitamin D manufacturing, sunlight can 'energize' our T cells. These immune cells must be able to move swiftly to the site of infection, and researchers have found that low levels of blue light in the sun's rays facilitate our T cells to move more speedily. However, in the UK and many other countries, it can be difficult to reach the daily vitamin D requirements during the darker winter months.

You can also consume vitamin D through the food you eat, and the best sources include oily fish, such as salmon, mackerel and sardines; eggs; and fortified foods, including breakfast cereals, dairy and spreads. This essential micronutrient can also be found in some mushrooms – one of my top tips is you can actually increase vitamin D levels if you expose mushrooms to ultraviolet (UV) light or sunlight. This is because UV light, especially UV-B, triggers the conversion of ergosterol, a naturally occurring compound in mushrooms, into vitamin D. Keeping mushrooms upside down on your windowsill can increase their vitamin D content. If you aren't a mushroom fan, then try chopping them up very small and adding to your meals. Or you could try a functional mushroom powder to get the benefits of these powerful myconutrients, which we look at in closer detail in Chapter 11.

However, as mentioned earlier, if you do decide to supplement, be aware that it is easy to potentially take too much vitamin D, especially if you opt for a high-dose vitamin D supplement or you take it for a long time. If this happens, you are at an increased risk of calcium building up in your body, and this may harm your heart, kidneys and bones. Therefore, it may be sensible if you feel you are at risk of being vitamin D deficient to speak with your doctor, who may suggest you have a blood test to confirm your exact levels. Then you'll know whether you should be supplementing and at what dose and for what approximate duration.

VITAMIN E

Vitamin E is a fat-soluble vitamin and a powerful antioxidant which helps protect the membranes of our body's cells from being damaged. Preventing and limiting damage is vital as damage may result in a dysregulated immune response.

This micronutrient has also been shown to regulate immune cell function, cell signalling, gene expression and metabolic processes. The mechanisms by which vitamin E may provide this protection include its role as an antioxidant and its function in anti-inflammatory processes and immune enhancement.

> **Vitamin E** has powerful antioxidant properties that protect our cells from the damaging effects of free radicals, which can damage cells and may contribute to the development of cardiovascular disease and cancer.[12]

In the UK, the current guidelines for adults aged 19–64 is that women aim for 3mg per day and men aim for 4mg per day. This recommendation should be fairly easy to meet, and if you consume a nutritious, diverse diet, you should be able to meet these guidelines. In the US, the recommendation is significantly different to that of the UK: for those aged 14 and over, 15mg is the recommended daily amount to aim for.

Foods rich in vitamin E include wheat germ oil, sunflower seeds, almonds, hazelnuts, peanut butter (no added sugar) and spinach. It can also be found, albeit in lesser amounts, in broccoli, kiwi, mango and tomatoes. For the average healthy adult, unless there is a confirmed deficiency, most people will be able to reach the vitamin E recommendation through their diet.

One of the main symptoms of deficiency is impairment of the immune response. However, some individuals who have coeliac disease or Crohn's disease, which are digestive disorders, may have impaired fat absorption. The digestive tract needs fat to absorb vitamin E, and people with fat-malabsorption disorders are more likely to become deficient than people without such disorders. Consequently, individuals who are affected by these conditions may have vitamin E deficiency.

Research has not found any adverse effects from consuming vitamin E in food, but if you do decide to supplement, it is imperative to avoid taking high doses of this vitamin as doing so can lead to some significant side effects, such as an increased risk of bleeding, nausea, diarrhoea, muscle weakness and fatigue.

It is important to note that vitamin E supplements have the potential to interact with several types of medications. So, if you do decide to supplement with vitamin E and you take other medications on a regular basis, it is advisable to discuss this with your doctor or medical practitioner.

VITAMIN A

Vitamin A is involved in many processes in the body and is vital for cellular communication, growth, development, male and female reproduction and immunity.[13] This fat-soluble vitamin also supports cell growth and differentiation, playing a vital role in the normal formation and maintenance of the heart, lungs, eyes and other organs.[14] It is critical for healthy vision as it's an essential component of rhodopsin, the light-sensitive protein in the retina that reacts to light entering the eye.

This important micronutrient is viewed as an anti-inflammatory vitamin due to its essential role in promoting immune function. It is involved in the development of the immune system and helps to support an active thymus, so it has both promoting and regulatory roles in the innate immune system and adaptive immunity. It can enhance immune function and provide an increased defence against multiple infectious diseases.[15] Vitamin A also helps to maintain the health of our gut lining as well as the lining of the respiratory system, which protects us against infections. It has powerful antiviral properties and helps to strengthen our cell walls and promote resistance to harmful viral infections.

The human diet contains two sources of vitamin A – preformed vitamin A (retinol and retinyl esters) and provitamin A carotenoids. Preformed vitamin A is found in foods from animal sources, whereas provitamin A carotenoids are plant pigments that include beta-carotene, alpha-carotene and beta-cryptoxanthin. The body converts provitamin A carotenoids into vitamin A in the intestine. Other carotenoids in food, such as lycopene, lutein and zeaxanthin, are not converted into vitamin A and are referred to as non-provitamin A carotenoids.

The daily recommended amount of vitamin A for UK adults is 0.6mg for women and 0.7mg for men. In the US, the recommended daily amount is different to that of the UK: for adults aged 19 and over the RDA is 0.7mg for women and 0.9mg for men.

Foods that are rich in vitamin A include liver, fish, eggs and dairy products. The majority of dietary provitamin A comes from leafy green vegetables, orange and yellow vegetables, tomato products, fruits and some vegetable oils. However, it is extremely important to highlight that liver is very high in vitamin A, so if you do eat liver or liver pâté regularly, watch your vitamin A intake, as if you're eating this particular food more than once a week, you may be consuming too much.

> The body may absorb up to 75–100 per cent of **retinol** and, in most cases, 10–30 per cent of beta-carotene from foods. Cooking and heat treatment can increase the bioavailability of beta-carotene from foods.[16] As with the other fat-soluble vitamins (D, E and K), you should eat vitamin A-rich foods with some fat to help your body absorb it.

As vitamin A is fat-soluble, the body stores excess amounts, primarily in the liver, and these levels can accumulate. Chronic hypervitaminosis A (regular consumption of high doses of vitamin A) can cause dry skin, painful muscles and joints, fatigue, depression and abnormal liver test results.

It is essential to highlight that vitamin A has the potential to interact with certain medications, so always check with your doctor if you plan to supplement with vitamin A and you take a medication regularly. Furthermore, research has demonstrated that supplementing with over 1.5mg per day over a long duration can impact bone health, which could increase your risk of fracture as you age. I would advise that if you are supplementing with vitamin A, keep to the recommended guidelines and consider your dietary intake.

Despite supplementing with other vitamins, pregnant women should avoid supplementing with vitamin A as too much can be harmful to the unborn baby. While vitamin A is very important for mum and baby during pregnancy, it is important to focus on getting the right amount from the diet during pregnancy.

VITAMIN K

The K in vitamin K stands for 'koagulation', which is the German word for coagulation and refers to the process of clotting. Vitamin

K activates a protein required for normal blood clotting, promoting wound healing and preventing excessive bleeding. Newborn babies are given a vitamin K injection to prevent a rare but serious condition of excessive bleeding since they are born with low levels of this micronutrient.

While vitamin K is primarily known for its role in blood clotting, it also plays a role in immune system function, regulating immune responses and reducing inflammation. Vitamin K's anti-inflammatory properties and its impact on immune cell function may indicate a potential role in managing autoimmune diseases, although more research is needed in this area. Some studies also suggest that vitamin K may play a role in regulating the gut microbiota, which in turn can influence immune responses.

The two main forms are K1 (phylloquinone) and K2 (menaquinone). They have similar functions, but it is thought that K2 may be absorbed more effectively by the body and stored for longer than K1. However, the body can also convert some of the K1 we consume into K2. K1 is mostly found in leafy green vegetables, such as kale, spinach and broccoli, and is identified by the NHS as the main dietary form of vitamin K. In addition, cheeses that are aged and high in fat have higher levels of vitamin K, with Camembert, Gouda and Edam all containing a decent amount.

Like vitamins A, D and E, vitamin K is fat-soluble, meaning it is absorbed best when eaten with foods containing healthy fats, such as olive oil, oily fish, nuts and seeds. When eating leafy greens, you may wish to consider adding healthy fats to your meal, such as a little olive oil on your salad, as this is a great way to aid vitamin K absorption.

In the UK, adults are recommended to consume approximately 1mcg of vitamin K per day for every kg of body weight. For example, a person weighing 70kg would need 70mcg daily. The guidelines are different in the US, where adult women are recommended to have 90mcg while for men the recommended daily amount is 120mcg.

Most people can meet the daily requirement through diet since vitamin K is widely available in the food we eat, so it is rare for adults in the UK to be deficient, although as we saw earlier some individuals may have a condition, such as coeliac disease, cystic fibrosis and ulcerative colitis, which could increase their risk of vitamin K deficiency due to fat malabsorption. Additionally, individuals who have had bariatric (weight loss) surgery may be at increased risk of vitamin K deficiency. Severe vitamin K deficiency can cause bruising and bleeding problems because the blood will take longer to clot. Also, bone strength may be decreased while the risk of osteoporosis is increased as our body requires vitamin K for healthy bones.

> Our clever gut microbes can also make **vitamin K** that the body can absorb.

Be aware that antibiotics can wipe out our beneficial gut microbes, and some of these bacteria make vitamin K. Using antibiotics for more than a few weeks may decrease the amount of vitamin K made in your gut and, therefore, the amount available for your body to use.

Vitamin K can be stored by the body, and the NHS advises that if you supplement with vitamin K, you should be cautious as too much can be harmful; however, supplementing with 1mg or less per day is unlikely to cause harm. If you do intend to supplement with vitamin K and take regular medication, speak with your doctor first as there are several medications that can potentially interact. Individuals who take blood thinners, such as warfarin, should not take vitamin K supplements without speaking to their doctor first and should also be aware of consuming too many foods containing vitamin K, as it may stop the medication working as it should.

HOW TO EAT FOR A BALANCED IMMUNE SYSTEM – MICRONUTRIENTS

The Minerals

Zinc, selenium, magnesium, copper and iron are particularly important for immune function as they support various aspects of immune cell development and antibody production as well as help fight off infections.

ZINC

Zinc is a mineral that is vital for immune system function because it supports immune cell development and communication and combats pathogens. It also helps protect our body's tissue barriers and reduces inflammation. This micronutrient is a powerful antioxidant and is required for enzyme activity as well as DNA synthesis. Zinc also plays a significant role in pregnancy as it helps to build a baby's DNA and cells. In addition, it supports a child's growth and development and is known for promoting effective wound healing.

> A **zinc** deficiency may affect your immune system's ability to function properly, resulting in an increased risk of infection and disease, including pneumonia.

Our thymus can shrink if we have a zinc deficiency, which then results in a reduced number of important T cells and potentially impacts cytokine production. This can lead to increased inflammation and oxidative stress. A mild zinc deficiency is more common than a severe deficiency but even a mild deficiency may affect immune function.

Zinc deficiency affects around 2 billion people globally and up to approximately 30 per cent of older adults. Plasma zinc concentration reduces as we age, and it is believed that this happens due to decreased absorption.

The recommended daily zinc intake for UK adults aged 19–64 is 7mg for women and 9.5mg for men. In the US, the recommended daily amount is slightly higher at 8mg for women and 11mg for men.

Most healthy individuals should be able to obtain all the zinc they need through a healthy, diverse diet. Foods that are rich in zinc include shellfish, red meat, chicken, turkey and dairy products, while plant food sources include whole grains, beans, nuts and seeds. It is important to highlight, however, that in some plant foods there are phytates that can reduce the absorption of zinc. This means that while plant food sources are still reasonable sources of this mineral, the bioavailability of these foods is less than animal products.

Research suggests that supplementing with zinc may help individuals who are already sick. Studies have also indicated that supplementing with small doses of zinc spread over the course of a day at 10–40mg can decrease the duration of the common cold significantly.[17] It is important to note that while studies and research have confirmed that 10–40mg a day can reduce a cold's duration, the Department of Health and Social Care in the UK advises that zinc intake should not be more than 25mg per day.

SELENIUM

This mineral also plays an essential role in immune health and is involved in antibody production. A deficiency can increase the severity or development of certain viral infections and can also impact both the innate and adaptive immune systems. It may also allow harmful pathogens to mutate, thus infecting for a longer duration.

Selenium has potent antioxidant properties and is vital for an effective immune response, managing systemic inflammation and supporting overall health. Selenium supplementation may reduce the risk and severity of viral infections and respiratory viral disease.[18] This mineral is also involved in supporting thyroid health and several studies have indicated that being deficient in selenium may actually trigger autoimmune thyroid disease. If you are deficient in this nutrient, then the thyroid can't make the required hormones.

Additionally, selenium is required for the glutathione peroxidase enzyme that plays a very important antioxidant role and prevents damage to the thyroid follicles. The thyroid cells can be damaged by harmful free radicals, which are a by-product of the body's biochemical reactions. It is believed that autoimmunity may occur when the thyroid cells are damaged, and because they appear abnormal, the immune cells then attack them, leading to further damage as well as inflammation.

> There is a significant association between **selenium** deficiency and coeliac disease. This deficiency is associated with malabsorption issues that are common in coeliac disease and can exacerbate inflammation and increase the risk of other autoimmune conditions.

Selenium is found in the soil and so is present in foods that are grown in the earth. Deficiency is quite rare unless you live somewhere that is known to have selenium soil deficiency. Selenium can be found in very high amounts in seafood, organ meats, sesame seeds and Brazil nuts.

The recommended daily selenium intake for UK adults aged 19–64 is 60mcg for women and 75mcg for men. In the US, the daily recommended amount is lower than that of the UK, and 55mcg is recommended for both men and women over the age of 14.

If you are considering supplementation, the most bioavailable form of selenium to supplement with is selenomethionine. However, whether you need to supplement with selenium depends on your unique and individual situation, so it can be helpful to discuss potential supplementation with a dietician or nutritionist.

> Supplementing with **200mcg** of selenium daily has been shown to reduce one of the main antibodies in Hashimoto's disease.[19]

MAGNESIUM

Our body needs magnesium, an anti-inflammatory mineral that is a cofactor in more than 300 enzyme systems which regulate diverse biochemical reactions in the body, including protein synthesis, muscle and nerve function, blood glucose control and blood pressure regulation. It is also needed for supporting immune health, regulating the immune response and regulating inflammation. Magnesium is also crucial for activating vitamin D in the body, and as we saw earlier, vitamin D plays a very important role in supporting the immune system. This essential mineral also improves the white blood cells' ability to seek out and destroy germs and pathogens.

Deficiency in magnesium can lead to temporary or long-term immune dysfunction.[20] Additionally, low magnesium can result in a cytokine storm, which is when the body attacks its own cells and tissues rather than fighting an infection. This can lead to increased inflammation, damage to our cells and tissues, a narrowing of our blood vessels and an increased risk of blood clots.

Good food sources of magnesium include leafy green vegetables such as spinach, legumes, nuts, seeds and whole grains. However, some types of food processing, such as refining grains in ways that remove the nutrient-rich germ and bran, lower magnesium content substantially.[21]

In the UK, the NHS recommends that for adults aged 19–64, daily magnesium intake should be 270mg for women and 300mg for men. However, the EU has a slightly higher recommended daily amount of 375mg. The US recommendations are slightly different: for adults aged 19–30, 310mg for women and 400mg for men is advised, while for adults aged 31 and over the daily recommended amount is 320mg for women and 420mg for men.

Those with gastrointestinal disorders may be at risk of deficiency as the chronic diarrhoea and fat malabsorption resulting from, for example, Crohn's disease and coeliac disease can lead to magnesium depletion over time. Those with type 2 diabetes may also be at a greater risk of deficiency as increased urinary magnesium excretion can occur in people with insulin resistance and/or type 2 diabetes.[22] Older adults are another group who may be at risk of deficiency. This is because older adults have lower dietary intakes of magnesium than younger individuals. In addition, magnesium absorption from the gut decreases and renal (kidney) magnesium excretion increases with age. Older adults are also potentially more likely to have chronic diseases or take medications that alter magnesium status, which can increase their risk of magnesium depletion.

Consuming a balanced diet will usually provide sufficient dietary magnesium; however, supplementation may be necessary in some cases, depending on lifestyle or medical conditions. Magnesium supplements are available in a variety of forms, including magnesium oxide, citrate and chloride. Absorption of magnesium from different kinds of magnesium supplements varies. Forms of magnesium that dissolve well in liquid are more completely absorbed in the gut than less soluble forms.[23]

The Department of Health and Social Care in the UK states that supplementing with 400mg or less a day of magnesium from supplements is unlikely to cause any harm. However, do not exceed 400mg per day as higher doses can cause diarrhoea.

COPPER

Copper is an important mineral for supporting our immunity and fighting infection. It is necessary for a series of physiological processes, including damage site repair as well as immune system function.[24] A lack of copper will lead to impaired energy production and affect the normal functioning of the immune system – and a dysfunctional immune response may lead to numerous inflammatory diseases, such as cardiovascular disease[25] and arthritis.[26] Increasing evidence suggests a link between copper deficiency and immune hypo-responsiveness as well as an increased risk of bacterial infection. As you can see, copper is critical for healthy, balanced immune functioning.[27]

A wide variety of plant and animal foods contain copper, and the richest dietary sources include shellfish, seeds, nuts, mushrooms, organ meats, wheat-bran cereals and whole-grain products. And it is good news for chocolate lovers – dark chocolate contains 70–85 per cent cacao solids, making it an excellent source of dietary copper.

Copper deficiency is uncommon in humans, with the average human diet providing approximately 1,100mcg per day for women and 1,400mcg per day for men.

As copper deficiency is uncommon, most individuals will meet the recommended daily amounts through consuming a nutritious and varied diet, so supplementation in most cases is not needed. Although if you are suffering from coeliac disease and you are concerned about copper deficiency, it is best to discuss this with your medical practitioner who can run tests to check if you are experiencing a copper deficiency.

> Approximately two thirds of the body's **copper** is located in the skeleton and muscle.

Adults in the UK aged 19–64 are advised to aim for 1,200mcg of copper a day. In the US, the recommended daily amount of copper for adults (both men and women) aged 19–50 is 900mcg a day. This recommendation is increased to 1,000mcg a day for women during pregnancy and 1,300mcg a day during lactation.

IRON

Iron is an essential component of haemoglobin, an erythrocyte (red blood cell) protein that transfers oxygen from the lungs to the tissues. As a component of myoglobin, another protein that provides oxygen, iron supports muscle metabolism and healthy connective tissue. This key mineral is necessary for physical growth, neurological development, cellular functioning and synthesis of some hormones. It is also essential for regulating both our innate and adaptive immunity so is crucial for a healthy immune system. Iron supports immune cell function and helps the body fight off infections, and a deficiency in this micronutrient can weaken the immune system and lead to an increased risk of illness.

Dietary iron has two main forms: haem (heme) and non-haem (nonheme). Plants and iron-fortified foods contain non-haem iron only, whereas meat, seafood and poultry contain both haem and non-haem iron.

Meat is recognized by most as being a main source of iron and haem iron is best found in sources of red meat. However, plenty of vegetarian-friendly foods are high in iron as well, including spinach, beans and even chocolate. Foods such as rice, oats, wheat, nuts, fruits and beans all have high amounts of non-haem iron. However, our body absorbs haem iron at an increased rate compared with non-haem iron, which means that individuals who follow a plant-based diet may not consume sufficient amounts of iron through their diet alone. If you are a vegetarian or a vegan, you should keep in mind that your body only absorbs 2–20 per cent of non-haem iron, whereas haem iron from animal-based sources has a 15–35 per cent absorption rate. Also, it is important to note that certain foods such as dairy products, eggs and fibre as well as tea and coffee can all interfere with the way you absorb non-haem iron and may reduce absorption. Fortunately, you can increase non-haem iron absorption from food sources by consuming foods that are rich in vitamin C at the same time.

By consuming a varied diet, you should be able to get all the iron your body needs; however, certain groups, such as infants, young children, teenage girls, pregnant women and premenopausal women, are at a greater risk of obtaining insufficient amounts and may be more susceptible to becoming deficient in iron. Iron deficiency progresses from depletion of iron stores (mild iron deficiency) to iron-deficiency erythropoiesis (erythrocyte production) and finally to iron deficiency anaemia.[28] Anaemia is characterized by low haemoglobin concentrations and reductions in haematocrit (the proportion of red blood cells in blood by volume) and mean corpuscular volume (a measure of erythrocyte size).

In the UK, the recommended daily amount of iron is 14.8mg for women aged 19–49, which reduces to 8.7mg for women aged 50 and over. However, women having periods after the age of 50 may need the same amount of iron as women aged 19–49. Also, it is important to note that women who lose a lot of blood during their monthly period are at a greater risk of iron deficiency anaemia and may need to take iron supplements. If you are experiencing heavy periods, you may wish to have your iron levels tested to check if they are adequate. The recommended daily amount of iron for men aged 19 and over is 8.7mg.

The US recommendations are again different, and for women aged 19–50 the recommended daily amount of iron is 18mg, which then reduces to 8mg for women aged 51 and older. For women who are pregnant the recommended amount is 27mg, and 9mg during lactation. For men the recommended daily amount of iron is 8mg.

As with everything immune and health related, too much can be as detrimental to health as too little. Both iron deficiency and iron toxicity can influence the functioning of the innate and adaptive arms of the immune system. While iron is an essential mineral for your body, increasing your absorption of haem iron significantly can cause a few issues. Too much iron can lead to problems like inflammation and even DNA damage because of the production of a dangerous free radical known as hydroxyl.

Thus, we need to ensure sufficient dietary iron intake while keeping to the recommended dietary guidelines. If you do supplement with iron, make sure you adhere to the recommended amount as you can experience some unpleasant symptoms, such as nausea, vomiting, gastrointestinal discomfort and constipation, if you take high doses of over 20mg. The NHS states that taking 17mg or less a day of iron supplements is unlikely to cause any harm, and if you are taking a higher dose as advised by a GP, do continue to follow your doctor's guidance.[29]

> Very high doses of **iron** can be fatal, particularly if taken by children, so always keep iron supplements out of the reach of children.

It is important to note that iron can interact with certain medications, and some medications can have an adverse effect on iron levels. Levothyroxine (also known as Levothroid, Levoxyl, Synthroid, Tirosint, and Unithroid) is used to treat hypothyroidism (underactive thyroid), goitre and thyroid cancer. The simultaneous ingestion of iron and levothyroxine may potentially result in a significant decrease in levothyroxine efficacy in some individuals.[30] Therefore, if you are taking medications, it is essential to discuss with your doctor before taking any supplements.

Summary

Numerous different vitamins and minerals are required for healthy immunity as these essential micronutrients each play a specific role in the immune response. Even a slight deficiency in one of these important micronutrients can have a profound impact on immune function as well as overall health. The easiest and best way to achieve the daily requirements of these key vitamins and minerals is to concentrate on eating a diverse diet. Focus on consuming a wide range of foods, including colourful fruits and vegetables as well as legumes, nuts and seeds. A varied diet will ensure that all the different components of the immune system receive the building blocks they need in order to function properly. Eating a diverse diet will also support our gut microbiome, which, as we know, plays a crucial role in immunity.

CHAPTER 9

Love Your Liver

The liver is located predominantly in the upper-right portion of the abdomen, although part of the liver is also located in the upper-left abdomen. On average, it weighs approximately 1.4–1.6kg in adulthood and is about the size of a football. This organ has several important functions in the body and is essential for the production of proteins, metabolism of nutrients and clearance of toxins. One of the major functions of the liver is related to innate immunity.

The liver contains the largest macrophage population in the body, and these essential immune cells play a vital role in destroying infectious bacteria and other harmful organisms that enter our body. They are also busy clearing cellular debris and wound healing. The liver also contains the largest population of natural killer (NK) cells in the body, which identify and eliminate cells that are infected with viruses or are cancerous. NK cells can also influence the activity and development of other immune cells, thereby contributing to both innate and adaptive immunity.

It is clear that the liver plays a vital role in immune function, acting as a key frontline defence against pathogens and toxins. It is ideally positioned to recognize pathogens entering the body via the gut, and appears designed to detect, capture and destroy bacteria and viruses.[1] As our adaptive immune system detects and starts to mount a response over days, our liver responds in seconds, holding the fort until the cavalry arrives.

> Our **liver** houses a significant number of **immune cells**, including phagocytes, the cells that engulf and destroy harmful invaders. It also filters blood, removing harmful substances and pathogens that enter the body, especially from the digestive system.

One of the main features of the immune system is 'immune tolerance', which ensures that the body does not harm its own tissues. This essential organ produces proteins that are crucial for immune function and helps to maintain immune tolerance, preventing excessive immune responses against harmless substances like food antigens. Although the liver's default immune status is anti-inflammatory or immunotolerant, under the right conditions it is able to mount a rapid and robust immune response when needed. Therefore, the balance between immunity and tolerance is vital to liver function.

This balance between immune tolerance and effective immune screening is maintained by interactions between numerous immune cells that are located in and recruited into the liver. If an inappropriate immune response disturbs this delicate balance, then autoimmune liver pathologies can develop. Additionally, the inability to launch an effective immune response may result in chronic viral infections or failure to clear cancer cells.[2] This function of the liver in maintaining immune responses and tolerance demonstrates the importance of the liver as an extremely important immune organ. When there is excessive inflammation present, even in the absence of infection, this may result in liver injury and tissue damage.

However, the liver is an incredible organ, and it has the ability to regenerate, which means that after an injury or surgery to remove tissue, the liver tissue can grow back to a certain extent. The liver tissue begins to grow back by having the existing cells enlarge and then new liver cells begin to multiply. Research indicates that within one week after removing two thirds of the liver, the liver can return to the same weight it was before surgery!

It is evident that the liver is essential to the body's metabolic, detoxification and immune system functions. Damage to the liver can impair its ability to filter toxins, produce immune-related proteins and effectively manage immune responses, making individuals more susceptible to infections. Supporting your liver through a balanced diet, regular exercise and moderate alcohol consumption while maintaining a healthy weight and avoiding toxins, as much as possible, is crucial for a strong and balanced immune system.

Autoimmune Disease and Toxin Exposure

Toxins are substances that, when they are ingested, inhaled or come into contact with your skin, can cause the immune system to react as the substance is deemed to be harmful. Toxins can also impact cells directly, causing damage and putting a lot of stress on your liver, which we know plays a key role in clearing toxins from your body.

Some examples of toxins include:

- paint
- petrol and diesel
- tobacco smoke
- household cleaning products
- glue
- compounds found in plastic, such as BPA
- heavy metals, including mercury, arsenic, lead and cadmium, which can be found in our food, water, air, dental amalgams and cosmetics.

Substances such as mercury, aluminium, dioxin, pesticides, asbestos, trichlorethylene and many other industrial and environmental toxins have been associated with autoimmunity.[3] These chemicals can lead to oxidative stress, T cell dysregulation and alterations of our immune cell messenger systems.[4] This can significantly impact our body's ability to mount appropriate and effective immune responses. Additionally, exposure to toxins can trigger inflammation, damage DNA, alter the gut microbiome and cause epigenetic changes – all of which can disrupt the immune system's normal function and lead to an inappropriate immune response.

The global increase in autoimmune disease prevalence and incidence rates corresponds with environmental toxic load exposure in people living in industrialized countries.[5] Many epidemiological studies have reported environmental factors to be key in this significant increase.[6]

> Several mechanisms may cause **immune dysregulation** and autoimmune reactivity, including toxic chemical exposure and genetic susceptibility.

Studies with twin subjects have determined that genetics can only account for an increased risk of autoimmune diseases and that an environmental trigger is required to 'switch on' the genetic expression of these diseases. Environmental chemicals may be a key factor in the onset of autoimmunity in individuals who are most at risk, and every single day, we are exposed to many different toxic chemicals: constant organic pollutants, toxic metals, solvents and endocrine disruptors are ever-present in our food, household and personal hygiene products, and even in the air we breathe. In addition, mould exposure can lead to the production of mycotoxins, which can disrupt immune function and potentially trigger autoimmune reactions, as can exposure to asbestos, which has been linked to an increased prevalence of systemic autoimmune disease.

Moreover, toxic chemicals deplete important, health-promoting antioxidants, such as the 'master' antioxidant, glutathione, and this can contribute to immune dysregulation and deterioration of immune barriers, including the blood–brain barrier and the intestinal barrier. The combination of these physiological changes and genetic susceptibility may lead to the development of autoimmune disease.

> **Glutathione** is known as the master antioxidant due to its crucial role in protecting cells from oxidative stress and damage caused by free radicals. It is a powerful antioxidant naturally produced in the body and is composed of three amino acids, namely glycine, cysteine and glutamate.

The term 'toxic load' is used to measure the amount of toxins in your cells and tissues and can also measure how long and how great your exposure to toxins has been. A toxic load can put significant strain on both the liver and the immune system, and when the liver is overloaded, it can lead to inflammation and impaired function and affect overall health. It also negatively impacts immunity and can cause immune function to become dysregulated, which may potentially lead to a greater susceptibility to infections and autoimmune responses.

The Danger of Heavy Metals

Heavy metals are non-biodegradable materials that exist in food, such as fruits and vegetables, dust, soil, air and water. Heavy metals are abundant in the environment, and exposure to them is becoming increasingly prevalent.[7] Diet is one of the main causes of human exposure to heavy metals since they are released into water and soil, accumulating in plant foods, including cereals, rice, wheat, roots and mushrooms, as well as animal foods, including fish, crustaceans and molluscs.[8]

These heavy metals can enter our bodies through the respiratory, cutaneous and gastrointestinal pathways and then accumulate in different organs, leading to their encountering various parts of the body, including the immune system. These metals are described as 'heavy' as they stay in the body, hiding away in our adipose tissue, which is basically our fat cells. They are difficult to eliminate, and this makes them similar to fat-soluble toxins. Our body fat attempts to protect our organs by trapping certain substances, including some heavy metals, allowing them to remain. This may be one reason why, when weight loss occurs, detoxification of heavy metals can also ensue, as our fat cells get smaller and, subsequently, release stored toxins.

The build-up of heavy metals in the body can have a significant negative impact on human health. Heavy metal toxicity can lead to decreased mental and central nervous function as well as damage to the vital organs, such as the liver, heart, endocrine glands and kidneys. Long-term exposure to heavy metals may lead to significant physical, muscular and neurological degenerative processes.

In addition, the interaction of heavy metals with the immune system may lead to immunosuppression or immunodysregulation and may have significant consequences for allergy or autoimmunity. While susceptibility to autoimmunity is determined by both heritable traits and environmental factors, research suggests that exposure to heavy metals may play a significant role in initiation and/or progression of autoimmune diseases.[9] Heavy metals can also cause alterations to our gut microbiota composition and function. They can disturb the balance of the gut microbiota, resulting in dysbiosis and other potential health effects.[10]

It is quite impossible to entirely avoid heavy metal exposure since these metals are natural elements that are present in the food supply, water and ground. Over time they can accumulate within bodily tissues, often without us even knowing that this is happening. Also, as heavy metal toxicity symptoms mimic those related to ageing – for instance, loss of memory, increased tiredness and muscle weakness – many individuals interpret getting older as the reason for their adverse symptoms, unaware that heavy metal exposure may be a significant contributing factor.

Heavy metals in foods, such as arsenic, cadmium and lead, have been associated with several different cancers, including lung, kidney, bladder, stomach, brain, skin, liver, prostate, renal, breast, pancreatic and endometrial cancers. They are also linked with an increased risk of reproductive, neurological, kidney, respiratory, skin, cardiovascular, immunological and developmental issues. These heavy metals can sneak their way into the foods we consume, and research has shown some chocolate, particularly dark chocolate, contains concerning levels of lead and cadmium. These heavy metals can be present in cocoa beans and potentially contaminate the final chocolate product through various stages of processing.

Some of the most common symptoms that often present in individuals with heavy metal toxicity include:

- cognition issues and brain fog
- low mood
- anxiety

- dementia
- tremors
- digestive disorders, such as IBS
- aches
- impaired vision, hearing and speech
- skin issues
- anaemia
- autoimmunity.

Let's take a closer look at three of the most common heavy metals.

MERCURY

Mercury is a naturally occurring element which is found in air, water, soil and the earth's crust. It is released into the environment through volcanic activity, weathering of rocks and human activity. Human activity is the leading cause of mercury releases, particularly coal-fired power stations, residential coal burning for heating and cooking, industrial processes, waste incinerators and mining for mercury, gold and other metals.

Once mercury is in the environment it can be transformed by bacteria into methylmercury. Methylmercury then bioaccumulates (bioaccumulation occurs when an organism contains higher concentrations of the substance than do the surroundings) in fish and shellfish. Large predatory fish, such as swordfish, king mackerel and bigeye tuna, are more likely to have high levels of mercury as they consume smaller fish that have also consumed the toxin. Fish with the lowest mercury levels include sardines, salmon, anchovies and trout.

All humans are exposed to some level of mercury. Unfortunately, mercury exposure can cause serious health problems and exert toxic effects on the nervous, digestive and immune systems, as well as on our lungs, kidneys, skin and eyes. It is considered by the World Health Organization as one of the top ten chemicals of major public health concern and is a particular threat to the development of a baby in utero and early in life.

Long-term low-level exposure to mercury can cause many unpleasant symptoms, such as short-term memory loss, low mood, gum disease, tremors, tiredness, sleep issues and anorexia. It can also impact the central nervous system and lead to tingling and numbness. In addition, balance can be affected, and it can cause hearing and vision changes. Mercury exposure increases the risk of autoimmune disease, and research has confirmed that individuals with the greatest mercury exposures have a higher risk of autoimmune thyroid disease as the mercury accumulates in the thyroid gland.

ARSENIC

Arsenic is a metal element that is widely distributed in soil, rocks, air and water. It may also be found as a compound where it is combined with other elements, such as with oxygen to form arsenic trioxide.

Arsenic occurs naturally in the environment so we can be exposed by breathing air and from consuming contaminated food or water. Fortunately, in the UK, arsenic levels are tightly controlled and exposures to arsenic in water, air and food are decreased to the lowest practical level to limit potential health risks.

> Certain places, such as Hungary, Bangladesh, West Bengal in India and Taiwan have naturally high levels of **arsenic** in drinking water.

Food is the most significant source of exposure for most people in the general population, with most arsenic in the UK diet coming from fish. The form of arsenic compound found in fish, called organic arsenic, is much less harmful than most forms used industrially, which are mostly inorganic. Please note that there is no evidence that eating fish poses a health risk from arsenic.

For the general population, inhalation typically represents a minor route of exposure to inorganic arsenic. In addition, individuals who sand or burn wood that has been preserved with inorganic arsenic may inhale released arsenic. Workplace exposure may also occur where arsenic is used or released, such as in metal smelting plants. However, there are compulsory safe limits in place to protect employees which are below the levels that are believed to be harmful.

> **Cigarette smoke** contains a large amount of arsenic, and smoking can double the amount taken in per day. Arsenic has also been found in some traditional medicines and herbal supplements as well as in cosmetics.

The International Agency for Research on Cancer classified arsenic and its compounds as being cancer-causing chemicals, with long-term exposure to arsenic increasing the risk of lung, skin and bladder cancer.[11]

Research reports that chronic exposure to arsenic has the potential to impair vital immune responses that could lead to increased risk of infections and chronic diseases. Arsenic can alter the activity of both our innate and adaptive immune cells, including lymphocytes, macrophages and dendritic cells, with studies suggesting that arsenic can impair the development, activation, proliferation and function of immune cells and lead to immunosuppression. It may contribute to autoimmune diseases, and while research has reported potential links between arsenic exposure and immune system dysfunction, more research is warranted to fully understand the complex mechanisms involved and the long-term health consequences of arsenic exposure.

MICROPLASTICS

While not a heavy metal, microplastics may also impact our immune and gut health. Microplastics are very small pieces of plastic that can take hundreds or even thousands of years to break down. Microplastics can enter the environment from several sources, including from larger pieces of plastic waste that are already in the environment and breaking down over time – for example, microscopic fragments from car tyres as they wear down, threads and microfibres of synthetic clothing, such as polyester, from washing machines, and waste directly from industry.

> **Microplastics** are found in concentrations **60 times higher** indoors than outdoors. We are constantly inhaling microplastics from our home environment as they are found in synthetic carpets, bedding, children's toys, water bottles and even nail polish.

Nowadays, plastic is ever-present in all areas of the environment: it is in the air, water and soil. It is used in most food packaging and is used for many of the foods we eat daily, such as dairy products, meat and fish, and drinks, including mineral water. Data from animal studies have shown that once absorbed, plastic microparticles can travel to the liver, spleen, heart, lungs, thymus, reproductive organs, kidneys and even the brain as they can cross the blood–brain barrier. In addition, microplastics can act as carriers of heavy metals.[12] Though research in this area is in its infancy, early research has indicated that microplastics may disrupt the delicate balance of the gut microbiome, which plays a crucial role in immune system development and function. This disruption can subsequently lead to inflammation and increased susceptibility to various diseases.

Microplastics can be engulfed by immune cells, which may result in increased oxidative stress as well as cellular changes. This can trigger the release of pro-inflammatory cytokines, potentially contributing to chronic inflammation and even promoting tumour development. Microplastics can also interfere with immune-related receptors and signalling pathways, particularly in the liver and spleen, thereby impairing the body's ability to mount an effective immune response. Research is ongoing, but there is an increasing concern that long-term exposure to microplastics could lead to chronic health conditions, including potential immune-related disorders and metabolic issues. As yet, due to a lack of data in this area, we don't have a full picture of the potential toxicity that microplastics may have on human health or the safety threshold for the human body. However, since plastic takes a long time to degrade and with more plastic continuing to be produced, it is highly likely that concentrations of microplastic in the environment will rise over time, increasing the potential for harm to both our health and the environment.

There are lots of ways that you can reduce your exposure to microplastics, such as:

- investing in reusable shopping bags, water bottles, coffee cups and food storage containers

- opting for glass or stainless-steel alternatives when possible
- reducing consumption of ultra-processed foods as these often contain higher levels of microplastics
- avoiding heating food in plastic as heat can cause plastics to leach microplastics into food
- avoiding plastic tea bags as many tea bags contain plastic that can release microplastics when brewed
- choosing loose fresh produce over packaged produce
- opting for clothing made from natural materials like cotton, linen or silk – buying second-hand can be a great idea
- washing clothes less frequently as washing clothes, especially synthetic fabrics, can release microplastics into the water, which then gets ejected from our homes into the environment and potentially back into the food chain
- using a laundry bag for synthetic clothes as this can help reduce the amount of microplastics released during washing.

How To Optimize Detoxification

How are toxins removed from the body? There are numerous evidence-based ways you can help to support the health of your liver and optimize heavy metals detoxification capability.

Eat a Diverse and Nutritious Diet

If you suspect you may be suffering from heavy metal toxic load, then I recommend eating a highly nutritious diet to optimize detoxification.

Focus on including:

- **Vitamin C-rich foods** – e.g. fruits (kiwi, berries, oranges) and vegetables (broccoli, pepper, kale). Vitamin C can help reduce the damage caused by heavy metal toxicity by acting as an antioxidant.
- **Sulphur-rich foods** – e.g. garlic and onions. This nutrient helps your liver detoxify itself of heavy metals like lead and arsenic.
- **Omega-3-rich foods** – e.g. flaxseeds and chia seeds. Omega-3 fatty acids can help reduce inflammation.
- **Bone broth** – This food may be helpful as it supports liver health by providing glutathione. It also contains amino acids that help support gut health.
- **Herbs and spices** – These plant foods are packed with antioxidants and have anti-inflammatory properties that can help eliminate heavy metals. Use lots of different herbs and spices when preparing meals to get the most benefits. Some of my favourites to use are turmeric, cinnamon, ginger, basil, oregano, rosemary, parsley and thyme.

Meanwhile, try to reduce these foods when detoxifying:

- **Potential food allergens** – If you suspect a common allergen (wheat, milk, eggs, soy, fish, shellfish, sesame, peanuts and tree nuts) may be causing you issues, try to avoid this while you are trying to support detoxification. If you are experiencing inflammation from a suspected allergen, your body will be under extra stress trying to detoxify from heavy metal poisoning as well.
- **Ultra-processed foods** – Often these foods are very high in chemical additives that may worsen your symptoms of toxicity and reduce your body's ability to detoxify.

> **Vitamin C, B1 and B6 deficiencies** are all associated with poor tolerance of heavy metals and an increased risk of toxicity.[13]

Prioritize Glutathione

If we don't have sufficient levels of glutathione, then we will have issues eliminating mercury as it can accumulate and damage our cells, leading to significant health and immune disorders. Individuals with low levels of this master antioxidant are unable to effectively eliminate the mercury that has built up in their tissues or which they have been exposed to. However, some of us have an increased risk of glutathione depletion due to our genes, and as we know, while we can't change our genes, we can control how they are expressed. This means that if you do have the genetic variation which causes your levels of glutathione to deplete very easily, luckily you can support your glutathione levels through your nutrition choices. In fact, you may have the 'ideal' genetic variation for optimal glutathione levels, but if your diet is deficient in the raw materials to make glutathione, then you can become low in this essential antioxidant.

> **Cysteine-rich foods** include chicken, turkey, yoghurt, egg yolks, oats, garlic and onions.

As we saw earlier, glutathione consists of three amino acids – glycine, cysteine and glutamate – with cysteine being the most significant amino acid as it contains sulphur, which attaches and binds to a heavy metal, such as mercury. We also need another powerful antioxidant, known as alpha lipoic acid (ALA), to help maintain our glutathione levels. The richest source of ALA is organ meat (liver, heart and kidneys), and it can also be found in red meat, such as beef, and plant sources, including spinach, broccoli, tomatoes, peas, Brussels sprouts and rice.

However, dietary absorption from plant sources does not deliver substantial amounts of ALA into the bloodstream, so you may wish to include organ meat or red meat in your diet. Organ meats are also packed with protein, vitamins and minerals, such as iron. Although, one important note to be aware of when it comes to organ meat – individuals who have conditions such as gout or haemochromatosis, or those experiencing vitamin A toxicity, should speak with a doctor before consuming organ meat. Pregnant women should also speak with their medical practitioner before consuming organ meat, particularly liver due to its very high vitamin A content.

Consider Coriander

Chlorella and coriander, also known as cilantro, may help detoxify some neurotoxins, such as heavy metals and toxic chemicals, including phthalates, plasticisers and insecticides.[14]

Coriander has been reported to be a potentially powerful antioxidant which can promote glutathione levels, which we have seen may be the mechanism for treating heavy metal toxicity.[15]

Activated Charcoal

Activated charcoal is a black, odourless, flavourless powder which has been used since ancient times to treat various illnesses and ailments. It has been processed to make it more porous and can be used in both a supplement and powder form. It may be added to various food and household products, such as toothpaste. As a treatment, activated charcoal works to eliminate heavy metals and toxins via adsorption, which is the chemical reaction where elements bind to a surface. In fact, it doesn't get absorbed by your gut and it reaches your gut in its unchanged form. Its porous surface has a negative electric charge that causes positively charged toxins and gas to bond with it, thus resulting in it attracting positively charged molecules, such as toxins and gases. When liquids or gases pass through this activated charcoal, they bind to it. These toxins don't get absorbed into your body; instead they get trapped in your gut and excreted through your stools.[16]

Activated charcoal is so powerful that it has been used as an emergency treatment for removing poisons from the body very quickly. It's full of carbon and can help discard heavy metals and other toxins.[17] It may be used to treat overdoses of both prescription drugs and over-the-counter medications like aspirin, acetaminophen and sedatives.[18] Research indicates that taking 50–100g of activated charcoal within five minutes of taking a drug may reduce the ability to absorb that drug by up to 74 per cent.[19]

If you want to try activated charcoal, opt for activated charcoal made from coconut shells or identified wood species that have ultra-fine grains. Also, it is important to note that when taking activated charcoal, it is vital to ensure you are sufficiently hydrated.

Hydration is also vital for optimal detoxification and liver support, as well as for immune and gut health. As with other essential 'nutrients', recommendations regarding water intake are available from various official bodies, such as the European Food Safety Authority and the Institute of Medicine. These recommendations generally range from 2–2.7 litres per day for women and 2.5–3.7 litres per day for men.[20] Therefore, when supplementing with activated charcoal, ensure you are drinking enough water per day to ensure sufficient hydration, and this will also help to prevent constipation and promote the elimination of toxins.

As with all supplements, I do recommend speaking to a qualified nutritionist, dietician or your doctor before taking activated charcoal. It is generally considered safe but may cause unpleasant side effects like vomiting, and may also interfere with some medications.

Limit or Eliminate Alcohol

Alcohol is the most frequently misused drug throughout the entire world, and in the United States it is the leading cause of liver disease. According to the 2024 National Survey on Drug Use and Health, 85 per cent of adults reported they drank alcohol at some point, while approximately 6 per cent confirmed heavy alcohol use, with earlier research suggesting that 10–12 per cent were heavy drinkers with alcohol use disorder.[21] Similarly, in other Western countries alcohol use disorders range from 7–10 per cent of the population. In the UK research indicates that around 21 per cent of adults regularly drink at levels that may increase their risk of ill health and disease.

Excessive drinking can severely impact the health of your liver and damage liver function due to the build-up of harmful fat, increased inflammation and potentially even scarring. If this occurs, your liver is unable to function properly and perform its vital functions, such as removing waste and other toxins from your body. Therefore, limiting or abstaining entirely from alcohol, is one of the best ways to support your liver and ensure your body's detoxification system is performing as efficiently as possible.

Sufficient Sleep

Making sure you get enough quality sleep every night is vital to support your natural detoxification system as well as your immune and gut health. Sleep encourages your brain to recharge itself, as well as allowing toxic waste by-products that accumulate throughout the day to be removed. As we will discover in the next chapter, not getting enough quality sleep is associated with numerous adverse health effects, including anxiety, high blood pressure and an increased risk of heart disease, type 2 diabetes and obesity.

Should I Do a Detox?

This is a question I get asked a lot! Detox diets are often advertised on social media with promises to help eliminate toxins to improve health and promote weight loss. Although the detox industry is booming, there is very little clinical evidence to support the use of these diets.

Additionally, they are not necessary as your body has its own highly efficient detoxification system. As we have seen, you can enhance your body's natural detoxification system and improve your overall health by consuming a nutritious diet which is diverse and includes plenty of health-promoting fibre and antioxidants. Also, reducing alcohol intake, ensuring adequate hydration, engaging in regular exercise and prioritizing sleep are all strategies that will help to support our liver health and keep our detoxification system in tip-top shape.

Summary

Our liver plays an essential role in immune function and is a key defence against any harmful pathogens and toxins. It also houses a significant number of immune cells, filters blood and removes harmful substances that enter the body, especially from the digestive system. Looking after our liver is vital for optimal detoxification and healthy immune function, and we can support this incredibly hard-working organ through simple lifestyle choices, including eating a balanced diet, ensuring sufficient hydration, engaging in regular exercise, limiting alcohol consumption, maintaining a healthy weight, managing stress effectively and avoiding toxins as much as possible. By adopting these lifestyle interventions, liver health will be prioritized, and a well-cared-for liver will lead to improved immunity and an overall healthier you.

CHAPTER 10

Sort Your MESS Out!

Mindset, Exercise, Stress and Sleep

Mindset

Major life difficulties and psychological stress can significantly impact immune health, decrease antiviral immunity, reduce resistance to infectious disease, increase inflammation and increase the risk of inflammation-associated disease.[1] Therefore, having a positive mindset and attitude is essential for a healthy, balanced immune system.

Studies have investigated the impact of negative self-evaluation and how it may affect immune responses. Negative self-evaluation can be described as a tendency to criticize and judge yourself harshly, and research has suggested that an individual's sympathetic nervous system response could directly impact how the body fights disease.[2] A negative self-evaluation could also affect a person's fight-or-flight response and lead to the body not conserving energy, resulting in the immune system losing both vital energy and strength, which we need to fight infection and disease.

One study also investigated the role of natural killer (NK) cells, which act as an initial line of defence against tumours and virally infected cells, and are also busy surveilling cells. Every cell reveals a code that the NK cells read, and if the correct code is not read, then the NK cells take this to mean that the cell is damaged; they then attach to that cell and destroy it. Looking after our NK cells is vital as they have been reported to be very sensitive to acute emotional stress.

> The **sympathetic nervous system** is responsible for the body's fight-or-flight response.

Loneliness

As social beings, our inherent need for social interaction, support and social stimuli should be met so that we can feel well and live a healthy life. In 1955, American psychiatrist and psychoanalyst Harry Stack Sullivan defined loneliness as an agonizing encounter, experienced when the need for human intimacy is not adequately met. However, in 1982, the former president of the American Nurses Association, Hildegard Peplau, described loneliness as when there is a mismatch between the quality and quantity of social relationships, those which we have and what we would like.

These definitions indicate that the reason for loneliness is not just being on our own but because we are not part of the social network or company that we would like to be. This suggests that feeling lonely and the actual state of social isolation are fundamentally different phenomena – loneliness can be inferred as an emotional experience while isolation is a lack of social contact.[3]

There are different types of loneliness:

- **Emotional loneliness** – When someone you were close to is no longer present, such as a partner, family member, close friend or pet.
- **Social loneliness** – When you feel you don't have a wide social network of friends, neighbours or colleagues.
- **Transient loneliness** – A feeling that comes and goes.
- **Situational loneliness** – When you feel lonely only at specific times, such as Sundays, bank holidays or the seasonal period.
- **Chronic loneliness** – When you feel lonely most or all the time.

Recent data suggests that loneliness has increased, particularly in the UK and US, and it can affect anyone, regardless of age, circumstance and background. Most of us will experience loneliness at some point in our lives, and it is a common misconception that only older people experience loneliness. In fact, it was reported that 16–24-year-olds are the loneliest age group in the UK.[4]

In the UK, **49.6 per cent** of adults (26 million) reported feeling lonely occasionally, sometimes, often or always.[5]

In 2022, approximately 7 per cent of UK adults reported experiencing chronic loneliness, meaning that they felt lonely often or always, compared to 2020 when 6 per cent of adults reported feeling chronically lonely.[6] Similarly, the US has seen a rise in loneliness and some researchers have declared it an epidemic.

To cope with loneliness, focus on connecting with others by

saying hello to neighbours, or making an effort to talk to friends or family – a simple phone call can make such a difference. You can also look for activities or groups that align with your interests, be that a sporting activity, book club, art class, language class or volunteering for a cause you care about. Spending time in nature can have a positive impact on your well-being and even a short walk outside can reduce feelings of loneliness and improve mood.

Having positive friendships has been reported to help us cope with stress and difficult life events. One study determined that having friends with us during a stressful time may help us see stress in a different way than if we were on our own.[7] The researchers' aim was to see if a psychosocial resource, in this case social support, can influence the visual perception of slants, and asked the research participants to evaluate how steep a hill was. Interestingly, those who had a friend with them estimated the hill to be less steep than those without a friend alongside them. Similarly, individuals who thought of a supportive friend during an imagery task perceived a hill as less steep than those who either thought of a neutral person or someone they didn't like. Both these findings suggest that the impact of social relationships on visual perception appears to be mediated by relationship quality, such as relationship duration, interpersonal closeness and warmth.

It has long been reported that loneliness has negative impacts on health and has been confirmed to affect the heart, potentially leading to coronary heart disease, stroke and metabolic syndrome.[8] Loneliness has also been shown to impact the brain, increasing the risk of poor mental health and dementia. In fact, studies confirm that individuals who report feeling lonely are more than twice as likely to develop Alzheimer's disease and other forms of dementia.[9]

> **Loneliness** has been shown to adversely affect glycaemic control, lipid (fat) metabolism, body composition, metabolic syndrome, cardiovascular function, cognitive function and mental health.[10]

Loneliness has also been demonstrated to be as harmful to our health as smoking 15 cigarettes a day! In addition, reported loneliness has been found to increase mortality of any cause, increasing the probability of death by 26 per cent. These findings strongly suggest that loneliness has a systemic impact on the body. It can also impact the immune system by potentially suppressing it while increasing the risk of inflammation, infections and disease, and even exacerbating existing health conditions. Loneliness can also affect antibody response against viruses and vaccines and immune cell activity.

Mind and Body Interaction

For strong and balanced immunity, mind and body interaction is paramount. Over the last three decades, mind–body therapies (MBTs), including tai chi, qigong, meditation and yoga, have received increasing awareness and attention from researchers aiming to elucidate the effectiveness and safety of these widely used practices. One meta-analysis looked at 34 studies and found that after 7 to 16 weeks of mind–body intervention, there was a moderate effect on reduction of the inflammatory marker C-reactive protein (CRP). Additionally, some findings suggested that mind–body therapies enhance immune responses to vaccination.

Tai chi, qigong and yoga are effective therapies involving moderate physical activity, deep breathing and meditation to encourage stress reduction and a relaxed state and may impact the immune system.[11] Meditation, including more mindfulness-based, stress-reduction exercises, has also been confirmed to promote emotional and affective responses to stress, and may impact the immune system even when no physical activity is involved.[12] Findings have indicated that MBTs provide many psychological and health functioning benefits, such as decreasing disease symptoms, boosting coping capability, regulating behaviour and improving quality of life and well-being.[13]

> **Mind–body therapies** decrease inflammation markers and can impact virus-specific immune responses to vaccination.

Alongside practising yoga for 20 minutes two times a week, one of my personal favourite strategies for improving mood and encouraging a positive mindset is, every day on waking, to think of three things I am grateful for; then, in the evening before bedtime, I write down three positive things that happened that day. This could be anything that made me smile; the last three positive things that I noted down were:

- Called my sister on her birthday and sang 'Happy Birthday' to her (badly!).
- My son won his school tennis competition.
- I wrote 2,000 words for my PhD thesis.

You can note anything at all that felt positive and meant something to you, such as meeting a friend you hadn't seen for a while, having a productive conversation with a new colleague or even getting a text message that made you smile. Or it could be something much more significant, such as getting your dream job, passing a test, getting a promotion or hearing that a friend is getting married.

Do give it a go as it is a very effective and positivity-promoting exercise.

Being thankful, grateful, counting our blessings and practising exercises of this kind have been used clinically for two decades. In 2005, the first study was carried out to see if we could use this method in our daily lives to boost well-being.[14] The study included 577 individuals who were randomly assigned to different groups. One group, as a placebo, were asked to write every evening about their childhood memories. Different groups were then given different interventions to try out, and one group of people had to draw up a list of three positive things that had happened and why they were positive. Over the next few months, all the research participants were given scales for assessing their happiness and the findings were notable. Within four weeks, the group who were assigned to note down the three positive things started to demonstrate increased happiness levels and a reduction in low mood and depressive feelings. Furthermore, these significant and positive results lasted for the six months of the study. On the other hand, individuals in the placebo group reported a short-lived increase in happiness in the first seven days, but then their happiness levels returned to baseline shortly after with no change at the follow-up six months later. Other recent studies have also shown that engaging in an intentional daily practice like gratitude journalling can improve sleep, reduce anxiety and help to support immune health. Just noting three things you are grateful for is so rewarding and literally takes 30 seconds!

Exercise and Physical Activity

The terms 'physical activity' and 'exercise' are frequently used interchangeably, but they are not necessarily the same. Physical activity is defined as any bodily movement produced by skeletal muscles which requires energy expenditure and includes exercise as well as usual occupational and/or domestic activity.[15] On the other hand, exercise is physical activity that we choose to do intentionally, which may involve aerobic (cardiovascular) training, high-intensity interval training (HIIT), strength training or resistance training. There is a vast and consistent amount of research that has confirmed the benefits of physical activity and exercise on health.

Regular physical activity decreases both the risk and severity of several chronic diseases, such as cardiovascular disease and type 2 diabetes, by improving heart health, blood pressure and blood-sugar control. It has also been shown to reduce the risk of various cancers, osteoarthritis and infectious diseases. The health benefits of physical activity are irrespective of age, sex, ethnicity or the presence of comorbidities. In addition, regular exercise and physical activity have been confirmed to benefit immune health, support recovery, combat inflammation and reduce the risk of infection.

A 2019 research review reported that moderate-intensity exercise can promote cellular immunity by promoting the circulation of immune cells, which helps your body detect infections earlier.[16] By engaging in cardiovascular, aerobic training at a moderate to vigorous intensity three to five times a week for 30 to 45 minutes per exercise session, recruitment and circulation of our capable immunity-defending cells is enhanced.

UK government guidelines recommend that adults aged 19–64 should aim for 150 minutes of moderate-intensity aerobic exercise a week as well as two strength-training sessions. Moderate-intensity physical activity can be defined as brisk walking, jogging, swimming or cycling. The recommendations are very similar in the US, where adults are advised to engage in at least 150 minutes of moderate-intensity cardiovascular physical activity a week as well as two muscle-strengthening sessions. Or, instead of 150 minutes of moderate-intensity exercise, trained individuals may wish to engage, over the course of a week, in 75 minutes of higher-intensity exercise, such as running, fast swimming or HIIT sessions. For some people, however, high-intensity exercise can be slightly too stressful and may increase stress hormones, such as cortisol, which then may adversely affect the immune system. Therefore, choose the most appropriate, sustainable and enjoyable cardiovascular exercise for you.

When it comes to strength training, two sessions a week is believed to be sufficient. We know how important muscle is for immune health as muscle tissue stores amino acids, which are essential building blocks for immune cells and proteins involved in fighting infection. During illness or stress, the body can break down muscle tissue to release these amino acids for immune system support, so protecting and maintaining our lean muscle mass is vital. In addition, muscles contain immune cells, including macrophages and T cells, that play a very important role in immune responses. Different strength training may include weight training, yoga, Pilates or even 15 minutes of body-weight exercises, such as press-ups, squats and tricep dips, which you can easily do in the comfort of your own home.

Regular exercise can delay changes in our immunity that occur as a result of ageing, which also helps to reduce the risk of infections. Immune dysregulation with ageing, as we saw earlier in the book, is referred to as immunosenescence. Increasing research findings indicate that engaging in regular exercise can improve regulation of the immune system, delaying the onset of immunosenescence. Additionally, in a study that included 150 older individuals aged 50 and over, it was confirmed that engaging in moderate-intensity exercise significantly reduced the risk of respiratory infection, such as the common cold or flu. The researchers reported that severity of infections decreased, too.

> **Habitual exercise** has also been confirmed to improve **immune regulation** and delay the onset of age-associated dysfunction.[17]

A sedentary and inactive lifestyle can contribute to a significant number of chronic inflammatory diseases as well as accelerate the ageing of the immune system. It increases the risk of cancer, chronic inflammation and infectious disease. Also, as we age and our thymus – which produces our important T cells – shrinks, we experience a reduction in immune function. However, physical activity engages our muscles and encourages the production of IL-7, a hormone that helps prevent thymic involution (the shrinking and ageing of the thymus) and allows our thymus to continue making T cells. Physical activity is also vital for our lymph to keep moving, which is imperative as it contains our important immune cells that need to get to where they need to be so they can protect us.

Research confirms that the immune system is very responsive to exercise, and physical activity is paramount for optimal immune health. However, in England one in four women and one in five men are confirmed as physically inactive, engaging in less than half an hour of moderate-intensity exercise per week! Moreover, just 24 per cent of women and 34 per cent of men perform strength training exercises at least twice a week.

In addition to the positive impact on immune function, physical activity supports gut health and promotes diversity of our beneficial gut microbes. Our beneficial microbes produce the health-promoting short-chain fatty acid butyrate, which supports immune health, and physical activity encourages our gut microbes to produce greater amounts of it. Recent studies also indicate that exercise and physical fitness diversify the gut microbiota, so physical activity can directly impact our gut microbial composition, leading to further increased improvements in gut health.

> The **immune system** and **gut** are inextricably connected, and when we exercise our immune system sends signals to our gut microbes, resulting in improved gut health.

One study determined that exercising for six weeks could significantly impact gut health. Participants followed a cardiovascular exercise programme for 30–60 minutes, which they performed three times a week for the six-week study duration. Analysing the participants' results at the end of the study, it was reported that their microbiomes had been affected, with some individuals showing a reduction in some microbes but an increase in other microbes. A significant number of participants showed an increase in the microbes that help to produce butyrate; however, after the participants went back to their original sedentary lifestyles for six weeks and their microbiomes were then analysed, it was reported that the microbiomes had reverted to how they originally were before the study. Thus, the beneficial effect of exercise on gut health may be somewhat short-lived, so regular physical activity is essential for maintaining optimal gut health. Remember that, like everything immunity and health related, we are aiming for balance. Excessive exercise can be as detrimental as too little exercise and can compromise gut function and cause temporary damage to the gut. It is thought that this occurs when our body temperature increases but blood flow decreases.

Athletes are particularly at risk of illness during periods of intense training and competition, so extra care needs to be given to immunity during these times. While undertaking intense training, athletes are also at a greater risk of inflammation, oxidative stress and muscle damage.[18] The wealth of acute illness research data collected during international competition events reported that 2–18 per cent of elite athletes experience illness, with higher proportions for females and those engaging in endurance events. Research confirms that athletes should ensure adequate carbohydrate intake for their needs, as a consistent finding is that carbohydrate intake during prolonged and intense exercise is associated with decreased inflammation as well as a reduction in stress hormones.

Walking is a great way to exercise and improve immune function and other areas of health. In fact, just half an hour of brisk walking can boost the circulation of NK cells and other immune cells. However, research shows that the immune cells return to the tissues they came from three hours after exercising; the immunity-supporting impact of exercise may be somewhat brief, so engaging in regular, frequent physical activity is key. In addition, walking has been confirmed to reduce the risk or severity of various health outcomes such as cardiovascular and cerebrovascular diseases, type 2 diabetes, cognitive impairment and dementia while also improving mental well-being, sleep and longevity. Walking's positive effects on cardiovascular risk factors are attributed to its impact on circulatory, cardiopulmonary and immune function. Meeting current physical activity guidelines by walking briskly for 30 minutes daily five days a week can decrease the risk of several age-associated diseases.

> **Cerebrovascular disease** refers to conditions that impact the brain's bloody supply. When the brain doesn't get enough blood and oxygen, the tissue can be damaged and die. Stroke, for example, occurs when a blood vessel in the brain becomes blocked or ruptures.

As older adults experience age-associated reductions in immune function, they are at a greater risk of severe illness and death from infectious diseases. During the Covid-19 pandemic, older adults were seen as a particularly vulnerable population because of their greater risk for serious illness and death from the SARS-CoV-2 virus. Subsequently, there has been an increasing interest in potential strategies to enhance immune function of older adults and promote overall health. This has resulted in walking-based interventions and exercise programmes being acknowledged as potential beneficial interventions for supporting immune function. Wide-ranging healthy ageing programmes that consist of walking-based interventions are key for boosting societal resilience to pandemics we may be faced with in the future as well as supporting healthy ageing for all individuals.

In addition to walking, low-intensity physical exercise can be highly beneficial for supporting healthy ageing, and this can be observed in the lifestyles of people living in the Blue Zones, which are regions of the world with the greatest number of centenarians. Researchers have determined five Blue Zones around the world: Okinawa in Japan, Sardinia in Italy, Nicoya in Costa Rica, Ikaria in Greece and the Seventh-Day Adventist community in Loma Linda, California. The lifestyles of the inhabitants in these regions have been analysed to investigate the factors – such as diet, social connectedness and physical activity – which are associated with their longevity and healthy ageing. A principal lifestyle factor of Blue Zone individuals is their high levels of physical activity, which in addition to low-intensity physical activities includes regular walking. Physical activity is an integral part of their day, and these populations will walk to work, or walk when running their daily errands. They also partake in daily gardening and other manual activities.[19]

> Numerous studies have investigated the research associating walking and physical activity and other lifestyle factors in the **Blue Zone** regions to healthy ageing and longevity.

In the Nicoya Peninsula of Costa Rica, physical activity is key as the region's terrain is hilly and the inhabitants tend to walk significant distances to work or to see family and friends. In conjunction with a nutritious, diverse diet that is high in whole grains, fruits and vegetables, the frequent and significant physical activity plays a major role in promoting healthy ageing in the people of Nicoya. Additionally, on the Greek island of Ikaria, where the terrain is rugged, individuals walk significant distances and are physically active in their roles as farmers and goat herders. Similarly, in Sardinia, physical activity and walking also play a crucial role in healthy ageing. As evident from the research surrounding Blue Zone populations, including walking and other physical activity in our daily life can be a highly effective intervention for healthy ageing and improving health outcomes in all individuals.

Stress

Stress can impact our immune health significantly and increase our risk of illness and disease. It is believed to be a main contributor to the onset of autoimmunity and research has confirmed that approximately 80 per cent of individuals with an autoimmune condition experienced a stressful event before diagnosis.[20] While acute (immediate) stress can temporarily strengthen immunity and encourage protection during infection, chronic (long-term) stress inhibits immune function. Chronic stress also increases levels of the stress hormone cortisol, which suppresses the immune response and increases inflammation. These unwanted effects can increase susceptibility to infections, worsen autoimmune conditions and impact the onset of cardiovascular diseases and other health conditions.

> **Stress** has been associated with exacerbating autoimmunity symptoms and worsening chronic inflammatory disorders, as seen in systemic lupus erythematosus, multiple sclerosis, rheumatoid arthritis and inflammatory bowel disease.[21]

On the other hand, stress-induced mediators, such as the brain chemical noradrenaline or glucocorticoids (steroid hormones that regulate immune response, inflammation and metabolism), can promote immune suppression, with glucocorticoids being used as an immunosuppressant for treating autoimmune conditions. These conflicting roles of stress on the immune system have led to much confusion, and as Hans Selye, the father of stress research, concluded, 'Stress is a scientific concept which has received the mixed blessing of being too well known and too little understood.'[22] This statement is still very current and can apply to the impact of stress on immune health as how stress affects immunity is still not fully clear. However, it has been well established that psychological stress and depression impair antiviral immune responses and activate innate immunity or markers of inflammation via effector pathways, such as the sympathetic nervous system (our fight-or-flight system) and the hypothalamic–pituitary–adrenal axis, also known as the HPA axis.

> The **HPA axis** is a complex system of interactions between the hypothalamus, pituitary gland and adrenal glands. It regulates our body's response to stress.

However, behavioural interventions, such as mind–body therapies, that aim to reduce stress and increase relaxation have been confirmed to strengthen antiviral immune responses and reduce markers of inflammation, particularly among older adults or adults experiencing high levels of psychological stress.[23] Three hundred studies which focused on stress and health were evaluated, and the researchers found numerous interesting findings, noting that in individuals who were chronically stressed for any prolonged amount of time, including a few days to several months or even years, every single element of their immunity was negatively impacted.[24] The researchers also discovered that older individuals, and those who were ill, were at a greater risk of stress-associated immune system alterations.

As well as impacting our immune health, stress has also been shown to harm our gut by altering the activity and structure of our gut microbiota as well as potentially being a cause of dysbiosis. Moreover, it can adversely impact the production of beneficial metabolites and increase the production of harmful substances. These stress-induced changes in our gut microbiota can significantly disrupt the gut–brain communication, potentially affecting mood and behaviour, and even contributing to mental health conditions. Some research has indicated that pro-inflammatory species can dominate at the expense of beneficial species in people with depression.[25]

> **Digestive disorders**, such as irritable bowel syndrome, frequently coincide with mood disorders and both may be indicative of a dysfunctional composition of gut microbiota and associated chronic inflammation.[26]

Stress appears to play a major role in altering the communication between our brain and gut, which can lead to increased inflammation, gastrointestinal damage, increased permeability and the condition leaky gut, allowing bacteria and their by-products to enter the bloodstream, potentially triggering inflammation and other health issues. In fact, one study that analysed couples whose relationships were in conflict and somewhat antagonistic observed increased gut permeability in these couples compared with couples who showed less hostile behaviour towards each other.[27] Although depression has been associated with increased intestinal permeability, this is among the first human evidence that chronic psychological stress, such as a disharmonious marriage, may be associated with leaky gut.

Furthermore, stress hormones, such as cortisol, can directly impact the types and amounts of microbes present in our gut. This can lead to a reduced number of beneficial bacteria like *Lactobacillus* and an increased amount of potentially harmful bacteria, as well as pro-inflammatory cytokines, metabolites, toxins and neurohormones, which may impact eating behaviour and lead to dysregulated eating. Gut bacteria may also increase stress responsiveness and increase the risk for depression.

Stress and depression not only affect our food and nutritional choices, but they can also change how we respond to food on a metabolic level. One study demonstrated that after consuming a fast-food type of meal, women who confirmed prior day stressors had increased insulin decreased fat oxidation and decreased resting energy expenditure compared with those who had experienced no prior day stressors. This is a significant concern for our metabolic health, as with a decreased caloric expenditure this may potentially lead to a notable 7–11 pounds of weight gain over 12 months.[28] This study illustrates the significant impact that stress can have on our metabolism.

It is imperative that we all recognize and determine what our individual stress triggers are and, subsequently, focus on finding and implementing the most effective stress-management techniques that work for us, as this can greatly impact our well-being. Fortunately, there are numerous evidence-based strategies that can help to manage stress, including meditation, yoga, physical activity and maintaining close and positive friendships.

Meditation

Meditation and mindfulness can often be confused. Mindfulness is defined as 'the awareness that emerges through paying attention on purpose, in the present moment, and nonjudgmentally to the unfolding of experience moment by moment'.[29] Mindfulness is a state of being fully present and aware of your thoughts, feelings and surroundings without judgement. On the other hand, meditation is a practice, often involving specific techniques used to cultivate mindfulness and other mental benefits. Essentially, mindfulness is the goal, and meditation is one way to achieve it.

One study confirmed the efficacy of the transcendental meditation technique in reducing stress and found the impact to be greatest in the participants who reported the highest levels of anxiety and stress.[30] The researchers concluded that overall meditation practice is more effective than most alternative treatments. Meditation has also been shown to benefit our immunity as it can enhance the number of certain immune cells as well as promote their function. Further promising findings report that meditation may have possible beneficial effects on specific markers of inflammation, cell-mediated immunity and biological ageing.[31] Meditation has been shown to also boost the function and number of certain immune cells, such as the NK cells and T cells.

One study conducted a comprehensive review of randomized controlled trials (RCTs) across 20 RCTs with more than 1,600 participants included. The researchers reported that a type of meditation described as 'mindfulness meditation' can modulate several select immune factors, appearing to be associated with a decrease in pro-inflammatory processes and increased cell-mediated defence parameters and enzyme activity, which protects against cell ageing.

Increasing research has determined that meditation can improve well-being and quality of life, and that regular meditation practice can decrease stress, anxiety and depression while improving overall mood, cognition, focus and sleep.

If you want to give meditation a go, then there are lots of great apps available to get you started, and you can practise meditation on its own or include it as part of your yoga routine, which we will explore in more detail below. Meditation involves lying or sitting on the floor, or in a chair if that is more comfortable for you. Alternatively, you can also practise meditation when you are standing or even walking. I highly recommend experimenting with a few different types of meditation on your own to see what you prefer, or you can also seek the guidance of a teacher who can help you establish a structured and consistent routine. Once you have created a meditation practice, I advise sticking to it for a few weeks instead of changing it too regularly.

Yoga

Physical activity and exercise, as we saw earlier in the chapter, are essential for a positive mindset as well as for managing stress, and yoga is an excellent form of exercise, for both the body and mind. The word 'yoga' derives from '*yuj*', which is a Sanskrit word meaning 'to join', 'to unite' and 'to yoke'. Essentially, yoga is a spiritual discipline that focuses on uniting the body and mind. The aim of yoga is self-realization, to overcome suffering, leading to the 'state of liberation' (*Moksha*) or 'freedom' (*Kaivalya*).

> **Sanskrit**, one of the oldest languages, is primarily known as the sacred language of Hinduism, and is also used in Buddhism and Jainism.

Yoga has been shown to decrease levels of the stress hormone cortisol and can decrease blood pressure and heart rate while regulating our breathing. It promotes mental and physical relaxation, which helps reduce stress and anxiety. Furthermore, the physical postures that are practised can promote flexibility, relieve tension and alleviate pain. And while certain yoga poses can help release physical blockages like muscle knots, they can also help encourage the release of negative emotions and tension. Yoga poses may also enhance the release of mobd-boosting chemicals known as endorphins, which can positively impact how you handle stress. Focusing on the present moment during yoga practice can increase your awareness, improve cognition and concentration, and focus your mind.

Numerous studies have confirmed the beneficial impact that yoga has on reducing stress and anxiety. A 2018 study reported that women who had practised Hatha yoga three times a week for four weeks experienced significant reductions in stress, depression and anxiety.[32] In numerous other studies, significant positive effects of yoga have been observed, including a reduction in stress, anxiety and depression. One study reported a greater improvement in mood and a more significant reduction in anxiety during 12 weeks of yoga intervention compared to the walking group intervention.[33] A second study confirmed the impact yoga has on controlling the mind and central nervous system, with researchers determining that yoga exerts a moderating effect on the nervous system, hormones and physiological factors, as well as regulates nerve impulses.[34]

Another study, which only included male participants without yoga experience, concluded that yoga decreased cortisol levels. It also reported an improved mental state in participants and observed a positive impact on parasympathetic nerve activity, which promoted feelings of relaxation.[35] Moreover, these factors were confirmed to be effective in preventing depressive psychosis and lifestyle-associated diseases.

In a later study, individuals who practised an 11-minute yoga nidra (yogic sleep) meditation for one month experienced a decrease in stress levels, an increase in overall well-being and an improvement in the quality of sleep.[36] Mindfulness, as a core element of the meditation, also increased during the study within the meditation group. The researchers also found that all the positive effects remained stable at the follow-up six weeks later. These encouraging findings suggest that just a very short dose of meditation can positively affect stress, sleep and well-being.

> **Yoga nidra**, or yogic sleep as it is commonly known, is an immensely powerful meditation technique. You lie in savasana (corpse pose) and the meditation takes you through the pancha maya kosha (five layers of self), which promotes a sense of wholeness.

Yoga nidra is an ideal option when you are too tired for an asana (moving through poses) or seated meditation practice, but you are keen to dedicate time to your yoga routine. I personally love yoga and have been practising for almost thirty years. Some of the most effective yoga poses for stress relief are so simple but highly effective. Here are a few of my favourite, easy and stress-relieving yoga poses.

CAT-COW POSE (*MARJARYASANA TO BITILASANA*)

This pose allows you to connect your breath to your movements as you calm your mind and release stress. Allow your breath to guide each movement.

1. Begin in a tabletop position: place your wrists underneath your shoulders and your knees underneath your hips.
2. As you inhale, turn your gaze towards the ceiling and allow your belly to move towards your mat, arching your back – like a cow.
3. As you exhale, draw your chin in towards your chest and bend your spine towards the ceiling – like a cat.
4. Continue to flow between these two positions for one minute.

CHILD'S POSE (BALASANA)

This pose helps create an inward focus and restore energy while supporting mental and physical relaxation. If more comfortable, place a cushion under your forehead or thighs.

1. From a kneeling position, place your knees together or slightly apart.
2. Sit back on your heels.
3. Hinge at your hips as you fold forward, resting your forehead on your mat.
4. Extend your arms in front of you or alongside your legs.
5. Allow your torso to sink into your thighs.
6. Breathe deeply and focus on allowing your body to relax.
7. Hold this pose for up to five minutes (you can start with two minutes and build up if needs be).

LEGS-UP-THE-WALL POSE (VIPARITA KARANI)

This is a very effective pose for promoting immune health as it stimulates lymph flow, provides deep relaxation and promotes healthy circulation.

1. Sit on the floor facing the wall, with your body as close to the wall as possible.
2. Lie on your back and place your legs up the wall with straight knees.
3. Position your hips next to the wall or a few centimetres away.
4. Place your arms alongside your body or place one hand on your stomach and one hand on your chest.
5. Hold this pose for 10–15 minutes (again you can build up to 10 minutes if needs be).

CORPSE POSE (SAVASANA)

During this pose, concentrate on breathing deeply as you quieten your mind and release any tension.

1. Lie flat on your back with your feet slightly wider than your hips.
2. Allow your toes to relax and turn out to the sides.
3. Place your arms next to your body at a 45-degree angle.
4. Ensure your head, neck and shoulders are aligned with your spine.
5. Breathe deeply as you encourage your body to completely relax.
6. Stay in this pose for 10–20 minutes.

If you can't manage yoga, then you can practise breathing exercises, known as *pranayama*. You can do this anywhere and it can really help encourage you to relax, regulate your breath and breathe deeply. This in turn helps to promote mindfulness, decrease stress, quieten your mind and calm your body. These exercises are very helpful when you may be facing an uncomfortable situation or negative emotions. If you are away from home or in work or have a busy day out and about, you can do breathing exercises by finding a quiet spot for a few minutes. I have done these exercises while sitting in my car for five minutes, and they are highly effective for calming your mind and body.

Meditation, yoga, physical activity and spending time and laughing with close friends have all been shown to be very effective stress-management techniques. We know how damaging chronic stress can be to immune and gut health, and that it can exacerbate numerous other health issues, so managing stress is vital.

Sleep

Sleep is an essential process for life, and we do it for approximately one third of our lives. It plays a vital role in our physical, mental and emotional health. Our sleep requirements and sleep patterns are impacted by a complicated interplay between our age, genes, behaviour, environment and social factors. Adults should sleep a minimum of seven hours per night to support optimal health.[37] However, studies have confirmed an increasing prevalence of adults who are having less than six hours of sleep per night over a long period.[38] This reduction in sleep is being experienced on a global scale, in low-income as well as high-income and developed countries, and sleep deprivation is an increasing worldwide concern.[39]

Why are so many people experiencing this increasing trend of sleep deprivation and reduced sleep duration, with nocturnal sleeping time below the recommended ranges for health? Researchers believe that besides medical issues, such as obstructive sleep apnoea and insomnia, factors including working hours; social demands, such as commuting, looking after children and caring for ageing parents; inadequate nutrition; smartphone addiction and anxiety are all at play in chronic sleep deprivation.

Worryingly, increasing research has confirmed the detrimental effect that sleep deprivation has on health, be that several weeks' sleep deprivation or even just one night of poor sleep.[40] Sleep plays an essential role in regulating our immune system and exerts an immune-supportive function, boosting our defence against infection and inflammation. In addition, sleep deprivation has been associated with changes in innate and adaptive immunity, which can lead to a chronic inflammatory state. This can increase our risk of infectious and inflammatory conditions, including cardiometabolic, autoimmune and neurodegenerative diseases.

> Just **one night** of sleep deprivation can reduce our NK cell activity by 30–70 per cent.

In the US, sleep deprivation has been associated with five of the top 15 leading causes of death, including cardiovascular diseases, accidents, type 2 diabetes, hypertension (high blood pressure) and cerebrovascular diseases (e.g. stroke).[41] Findings have also linked sleep deprivation to an increased risk of stroke, cancer and neurodegenerative diseases as well as low mood, depression and anxiety. In addition, sleep deprivation and disturbances are commonly reported in autoimmune diseases; however, immunotherapy in individuals with autoimmune pathologies has been shown to result in sleep improvement.[42]

> **Sleep** needs differ between people; however, the NHS recommends that healthy adults aim for between seven and nine hours of sleep, while children and teenagers require more, and a newborn baby will sleep anywhere between eight and 16 hours.[43]

Insufficient sleep impacts our endocrine, metabolic and immune pathways. Sleep deprivation may result in deregulated immune responses with increased pro-inflammatory signalling, increasing the risk for the onset or exacerbation of infection as well as inflammation-associated chronic diseases. Sufficient sleep is vital for healthy immunity and to promote a balanced immune defence against infection and inflammation.

Sleep deprivation also significantly affects gut health and can result in an increased risk of dysbiosis.[44] Research shows sleep deprivation can cause an increased Firmicutes:Bacteroidetes ratio while reducing microbial diversity and richness, which in turn can adversely affect the immune system.[45] This ratio change is considered a sign of gut dysbiosis and has been linked to metabolic issues such as insulin resistance.

> **Circadian rhythm** refers to our body's natural sleep–wake cycle and plays an essential role in regulating various physiological processes, including the gut microbiome.

Long-term disruptions to our circadian rhythm – whether through shift work or genetic mutations that impact the body's internal clock – can affect our gut microbes, impact microbial composition and increase the risk of dysbiosis; even jet lag can negatively affect the gut's microbial community. It can also result in increased inflammation and suppressed immunity. Circadian rhythm disruption can lead to even more issues, such as impacting nutrient metabolism and the production of beneficial metabolites, such as the super-important short-chain fatty acid butyrate. This can potentially lead to metabolic imbalance and increase our risk of metabolic diseases, including obesity, type 2 diabetes and non-alcoholic fatty liver disease.[46]

While sleep affects gut health, in turn our gut microbiome affects sleep, and there is considerable evidence demonstrating that the gut microbiome not only impacts our digestive, metabolic and immune functions, but it also regulates our sleep. In fact, preliminary evidence suggests that microorganisms such as our gut bacteria and our circadian genes do interact with each other.[47] In addition, research indicates that *Clostridiales*, *Lactobacillales* and *Bacteroidales*, which account for approximately 60 per cent of the gut microbiota, showed significant diurnal fluctuations, meaning that they peak and change at different times over the course of a single day.[48] So while one species of bacteria may be more abundant in the morning, another may be more plentiful in the evening. This suggests that the gut microbiome changes and fluctuates in a 24-hour period.

We all have very individual microbiomes with hundreds of species in different quantities, and our highly unique gut microbiomes can differ significantly at various points in the day. It could even potentially be suggested that alterations in our circadian rhythm through certain behaviour, such as shift work, flying and jet lag, could possibly lead to an imbalance of the gut microbiome and even impact metabolic health. However, more research in this area is needed, particularly in humans.

Stress is a significant cause of sleep issues, such as insomnia, and individuals with sleep disorders often experience increased anxiety. When experiencing stress, these sleep problems often worsen and result in negative impacts on our gut microbiota composition. The altered microbiota may then affect both immune and nervous system functioning, thus decreasing our ability to cope with both psychological and physical stress.[49]

> The **enteric nervous system** is the intrinsic nervous system of the gastrointestinal tract, often referred to as the 'second brain' due to its complexity and ability to function somewhat autonomously. It is a vast network of neurons (nerve cells) that control digestion, secretion and motility within the gut. It operates independently of the central nervous system but also communicates with it.

Fortunately, there are several very simple strategies that can improve our quality of sleep. One of the most effective strategies for improving sleep quality is to ensure you get morning sunlight exposure. This helps to regulate your circadian rhythm (your body clock) and signals to the brain that it is time to wake up and be alert. Morning light can switch off your brain's production of melatonin (the hormone that promotes sleep), and in the evening, melatonin will increase in response to the dark, to make you feel tired and ready for sleep. Sunlight exposure will also keep your vitamin D levels topped up, and research has reported that low serum levels of vitamin D are associated with an increased risk of sleep disorders.

Regular physical activity has also been shown to improve sleep quality and duration. One study analysed the impact of a 24-week, home-based, moderate-intensity walking intervention on various menopausal symptoms, including sleep, in 173 sedentary women aged 45–65.[50] The study reported that the frequency of adherence to walking played a significant role and was a predictor of a positive change and improvement in sleep symptoms. Additionally, in a longitudinal study (a research method that repeatedly collects data from the same sample over an extended period) that included 103 midlife women aged 40–60, greater physical activity levels during the day were associated with an increase in total sleep time at night, and this benefit was more pronounced in women who were overweight and obese.[51] A later study investigated the impact of walking on sleep quality and duration in 59 healthy participants with an average age of 49. The researchers acknowledged a positive relationship between daily active minutes and sleep quality, with women who were more active and did more steps experiencing better sleep quality than those who were not as active.[52]

Supplementing with an amino acid called glycine may potentially also help to promote sleep quality. Glycine is the main amino acid in collagen, which is the main structural protein of connective tissue, such as bone, skin, ligaments, tendons and cartilage. It helps to build proteins required for tissue and hormone maintenance as well as supporting heart and liver health, and it has been reported to decrease the risk of type 2 diabetes and help to maintain muscle mass. It has a calming effect on the brain and could help you fall and stay asleep by reducing your core body temperature.[53] Studies show that in individuals who struggle with sleep issues and are sleep-deprived, supplementing with 3g of glycine before bed may help to reduce how long it takes to fall asleep and promote sleep quality. It has also been reported to reduce daytime fatigue and enhance cognition.

Another study investigated whether a glycine-rich collagen peptides supplement could enhance sleep quality in physically active men with self-reported sleep complaints. The researchers reported that supplementing with 15g a day for one week with glycine-rich collagen peptides resulted in reduced nocturnal awakenings and improved cognitive function and performance. These findings indicate that glycine-rich collagen supplements could improve sleep quality in athletic individuals who are experiencing sleep complaints.

However, it is important to note that if you do decide to supplement with glycine and take other medications, you must check with your doctor before supplementing as glycine can interact with and decrease the effectiveness of other medications.

Other Tips to Improve Sleep Quality

- Engage in regular physical activity. However, make sure you exercise several hours before bedtime, otherwise it can make you feel more alert and lead to difficulties falling asleep as well as disrupted sleep.
- Limit caffeine after 12pm as this can cause sleep disruptions if you are sensitive to the effects of caffeine. (*Dark chocolate has caffeine and one small bar of approximately*

SORT YOUR MESS OUT!

30g may have as much as 20mg of caffeine, compared with 30g of milk chocolate, which contains approximately 6mg of caffeine.)

- If you are an afternoon napper, ensure they are short naps as longer naps will make falling asleep more difficult later.
- Keep to a regular waking routine – aim to wake at the same time each day, if possible.
- Don't eat late at night. This can affect sleep as our body is working hard to digest the food.
- If you smoke or drink alcohol, try to limit it in the evening as both can disrupt sleep.
- Create a relaxing bedtime routine that works for you.
- Having an Epsom (magnesium) salt bath can really help you to relax and has been reported to encourage sleep by reducing stress and helping to relax the muscles. Soaking in a warm Epsom salt bath before bed can promote a state of calm and aid in a more restful night's sleep.
- Turn off your phone and other electronic devices an hour before bed as the light from these devices can promote brain activity, which can make us feel alert and prevent us from falling asleep.
- Keep your bedroom at the ideal sleeping temperature (18.3°C/65°F) as too warm or too cold can both impact sleep.
- Invest in comfortable bedding, including a supportive mattress and pillows.
- Consider using earplugs to block out noise.

If you are experiencing persistent sleep problems, then consulting with a healthcare professional or sleep specialist is recommended as this can help you identify the underlying causes of your sleep issues, and the appropriate treatment can then be recommended.

Summary

A positive mindset, sufficient exercise and sleep, and effective stress management are crucial to achieving optimal immunity. It is very easy in this modern world – and with a huge number of our interactions conducted online and not in person – to feel lonely. However, loneliness can impact the immune system by suppressing it while increasing the risk of inflammation, infections and disease. If you are experiencing loneliness, try to make an effort to talk to neighbours, friends and family more, volunteer for a cause you are passionate about or maybe join a local walking group. Walking is great exercise, and spending time in nature can also have a positive impact on your well-being and reduce feelings of loneliness. A walk outside is perfect as it incorporates beneficial physical activity, improves mood and mindset, reduces stress and can also improve sleep quality and duration!

CHAPTER 11

Should I Supplement?

Along with 'What is the best way to lose weight?' this is the question I get asked the most – in fact, almost every single day. Some of the supplements I get asked most about include vitamin D, omega-3 fatty acids, probiotics and more recently myconutrients, which are medicinal mushroom products that can be found in the form of tinctures, teas and supplements.

My advice is to aim to get all your nutrient requirements through your nutrition and food, as every food is made up of differing amounts of macronutrients (carbohydrates, proteins and fats), micronutrients (vitamins and minerals), fibre and other important nutrients, such as phytonutrients (plant compounds). There are hundreds of different phytonutrients, and they have been shown to benefit immune health and gut health as well as neurological function. As we saw earlier, these powerful chemicals are found in abundance in plant foods, such as fruits, vegetables, herbs and spices, and are most likely found there in greater quantity and variety than in single- or multi-nutrient supplements. Certain foods that are fermented (sauerkraut, kimchi, miso) are also rich in probiotic bacteria that help keep our guts 'topped up' with beneficial bacteria, which is essential for good gut health. By including real wholefoods over supplements, we are consuming other nutrients which help to promote both nutrient absorption and bioavailability (the amount we absorb from the nutrient and effectively use in the body). These nutrients which help enzymes in our body carry out metabolic reactions include the B vitamins, vitamin C, vitamin K and minerals such as zinc, magnesium, copper and iron.

However, if you have a diagnosed vitamin or mineral deficiency, or you follow a strict vegan diet and you may be low in vitamin B12 (found in animal products), or you are ill or recovering from an illness and not up to eating anything, then nutritional supplements, I believe, can play a very helpful role in ensuring you meet your daily micronutrient requirements and support your health.

Again, it is all about balance and I advise that you should take supplements when you need them and to learn to read labels to understand the ingredients that are included. It is essential to see how much of a particular nutrient is included as toxicity (too much) is as bad as having a deficiency. This is because toxicity of a micronutrient can potentially lead to some very nasty symptoms and in some instances can be fatal. It is also important to check whether there are any harmful additives or fillers.

Check Labels for These Additives

If you decide to supplement, one of the first things to check is that the supplement does not contain any chemical additives, which may harm health. These potentially harmful additives can be found in cheaper but also more costly supplements, so don't be fooled into thinking the more expensive supplements are necessarily better. Why these additives are added can be for several different reasons, including:

- to bulk and bind the supplements so they stick together
- to make the supplements smooth or give a particular texture
- as a colouring agent

- as a flow agent, to prevent ingredients clumping together when being made or sticking to machinery.

> Not all **additives** are harmful – some can actually aid the absorption of nutrients.

Some of the additives to avoid include:

TITANIUM DIOXIDE

This is the one additive I recommend avoiding at all costs as it has been classified as a carcinogen by the European Food Safety Authority (EFSA). Titanium dioxide is the biggest no-no for your health: as well as being carcinogenic (capable of causing cancer), research has confirmed that it is associated with inflammation and genotoxicity (the ability of chemicals to damage our genetic information in a cell, resulting in mutations), and it also stimulates free radicals, which can cause damage to your body's cells.

The International Agency for Research on Cancer indicates that titanium dioxide has been used for decades by numerous leading brands to colour supplements white, and it is still found in many supplements, including high-end, expensive brands. Please do read your supplement labels to check for this additive.

In 2022, the EFSA banned titanium dioxide as an additive due to safety concerns. However, the Food Standards Agency in the UK has conducted its own review of the safety data and determined that there are no identified safety concerns. Therefore, titanium dioxide remains an authorized food additive in the UK and is allowed to be added to nutritional supplements. While it is still not banned in the UK, some manufacturers have started to offer products without titanium dioxide. However, some research suggests that it is included in more than a third of supplements sold online and on the high street, including high-end and premium supermarkets.

MAGNESIUM STEARATE

We know that magnesium is one of the most essential minerals required for our health, and it has become one of the most popular supplements. There are several different forms of magnesium, and magnesium stearate is a chemical additive which is a white, powdery salt composed of magnesium and stearic acid. It is very commonly found in supplements and is added to act as a lubricant, anti-caking agent and flow agent to speed up the manufacturing process. While commonly found in supplements, it has also been found in chewing gum, confectionery and even cosmetics.

Magnesium stearate can be derived from plant sources, predominantly made from palm oil, one of the biggest drivers of global deforestation, as well as animal sources, including pork fat, beef fat and chicken fat. Therefore, if you do take a supplement and follow a vegan or vegetarian eating plan, you may wish to check with the manufacturer about which source is included.

While some researchers have raised concerns about its potential impact on toxicity and bioavailability, the EFSA and the Medicines and Healthcare products Regulatory Agency have found no safety concerns for use in approved applications, including as an additive in food and supplements. However, too much magnesium stearate can have a laxative effect and may irritate the mucosal lining of the gut and cause diarrhoea. While rare, some people can experience a sensitivity or allergy to it.

SODIUM BENZOATE

Sodium benzoate is a preservative and a man-made compound used to promote shelf life and inhibit the growth of bacteria, yeast and mould. However, it can become carcinogenic when combined with vitamin C as it can convert to benzene, which is a known carcinogen. Also, preliminary studies have suggested a link between sodium benzoate and ADHD in children, cell damage due to free radical production, and decreased levels of the hormone leptin, which has an appetite-suppressing effect.

It is important to highlight that a significant negative impact is associated most typically with high intake of sodium benzoate, and while these findings are of concern, more research is needed to confirm them.

MALTODEXTRIN

Maltodextrin is a white, starchy powder that is used as a filler and is found in numerous supplements, including those produced by leading collagen powder brands. Some studies have suggested that maltodextrin can negatively affect our gut bacteria, and it can increase the activity of *Escherichia coli* (E. coli) bacteria, which have a role in the development of an inflammatory bowel disease known as Crohn's disease. It has also been associated with the survival of *Salmonella* bacteria, which may cause gastroenteritis (inflammation of the stomach and intestines, typically caused by a bacterial or viral infection) and chronic inflammatory conditions.

It has also been shown to cause gastrointestinal discomfort, such as bloating, gas and diarrhoea in some people. Some individuals can experience an allergic reaction to it, which can result in skin irritation, rashes, itching, cramping, difficulty breathing and asthma.

CARRAGEENAN

Carrageenan is used as a thickening and stabilizing agent, and also to enhance texture and ensure a consistent formulation. It has been linked to digestive issues, such as intestinal inflammation, irritable bowel syndrome and bloating as well as glucose intolerance, colon cancer and food allergies. However, it is important to note that most of the research conducted to evaluate the potential adverse impact of carrageenan has been on animals and cell cultures, and further research in humans is warranted to confirm these findings.

HYDROGENATED OILS

Hydrogenated oils, also known as trans fats, are used as fillers and can increase the risk of heart disease. Check the ingredients section on your supplement label for 'vegetable fat', 'hydrogenated' or 'partially hydrogenated' oils, as these can indicate the presence of trans fats, which are potentially harmful to our health. Some of these health risks include increased low-density lipoprotein (LDL) cholesterol, often referred to as the 'bad' cholesterol, decreased high-density lipoprotein (HDL) cholesterol, aka the 'good' cholesterol, as well as a greater risk of heart disease. Other research suggests a link between trans fats and type 2 diabetes, certain types of cancer and a lower birth weight in babies.

ARTIFICIAL COLOURS AND FLAVOURS

Colourings and flavourings are frequently used to improve the appearance of supplements, but some have been associated with hyperactivity, particularly in children. In 2018, the US Food and Drug Administration banned seven artificial flavourings, six of which were banned after research confirmed that they caused cancer in rodents. The six included benzophenone, ethyl acrylate, eugenyl methyl ether, myrcene, pulegone and pyridine. Styrene, which in 2011 had been determined by the US National Toxicology Program to be 'reasonably anticipated' as a carcinogen to humans, was the seventh flavouring to be banned.

TALC

Talc is used as a filler and anti-caking agent to prevent clumping, sticking together during manufacturing and damaging machinery. The EFSA has re-evaluated talc as a food additive and identified gaps in the data surrounding its long-term toxicity, carcinogenic properties and reproductive impact. It has raised safety concerns and its use is under scrutiny; while not currently banned, future restrictions or bans are possible.

ARTIFICIAL SWEETENERS

As we saw earlier, artificial sweeteners can have a significant negative effect on gut health, so I would advise limiting or avoiding, if possible.

> As yet, we don't know the effects of **chemical** additives, such as colourings and flavourings, when consumed in combinations every day for years. Therefore, we don't know the impact they may have on our bodies and health.

If you are concerned about a specific product, then you can often find more information about the ingredients that are included on the supplement manufacturer's website.

Reading Supplement Labels

As explored above, many supplements sold online and in leading shops can contain potentially harmful chemical additives. Be savvy when it comes to marketing claims, as just because a supplement says that it is 'natural', this does not mean it is free of potentially harmful additives. Therefore, checking supplement labels is vital.

When you check labels, make sure you look at the ingredients list, which is often in smaller print, written in a paragraph. It is a legal requirement that the ingredients list must contain *every* ingredient in your supplement, including the additives that are included. Don't just check the nutritional information table as this doesn't show all the ingredients used. A nutritional table only indicates the ingredients in the supplement that provide a nutritional benefit. Additionally, when you look at the nutritional table, make sure that none of the nutrients are at toxically high levels of a nutrient as this can potentially result in numerous significant adverse side effects.

I always recommend that you speak with your doctor or medical practitioner, especially if you are taking medication, before taking any nutritional supplement.

Immune-Supporting Micronutrients

While we covered the immune-supporting micronutrients in detail earlier in Chapter 8, I am going to touch on vitamin D and magnesium supplementation briefly in this chapter as data suggests that deficiency can be common in these two particular micronutrients.

We will then explore in greater detail other immunity-nourishing nutrients that you may be considering supplementing with.

VITAMIN D

Official UK guidelines have advised that everyone should be supplementing with 10mcg of vitamin D from October through to April. This is a guideline at population level, and it is not a personalized recommendation for each and every one of us. I have seen a huge number of people who have followed this recommendation and subsequently have been found to have dangerously high and toxic levels of vitamin D. This may be because some people may only need vitamin D for one or two of the dark winter months, for example. I would recommend, if possible, that you check your vitamin D levels with an at-home finger-prick test before you supplement with vitamin D to see if your current levels are normal or low and you would benefit from supplementation. This could also save you money in the long term.

As I mentioned on p. 143, Vitamin D is mainly synthesized through exposing our skin to the sun's UV rays, and as we store vitamin D in our bodies, we can actually 'bank' vitamin D from the sunny summer months. Depending on your location and available hours of sunlight, you may only need to supplement during the two or three darkest months of the year.

Do note that the water-soluble vitamins (the B vitamins and vitamin C) aren't stored in the body, so while an excess can cause some unpleasant symptoms and side effects, such as nausea, gastrointestinal discomfort, vomiting and headaches, they are not as much of a concern as our body can excrete excess of these vitamins in our urine. However, vitamins A, D, E and K are fat-soluble vitamins, and excessive intake of these can be a significant concern as they are stored in the body. Therefore, if you are supplementing with any of the fat-soluble vitamins, ensure that you are taking only what your medical practitioner may have advised or stick to 100 per cent RDI of that nutrient.

MAGNESIUM

Magnesium is a mineral that has gained a lot of media attention recently and has been described as the 'mineral of the moment' due to its wide-ranging health benefits. It plays a vital role in immune health and how our immune cells function, and it is also key for maintaining our gut health.

Magnesium deficiency is associated with several health issues, such as type 2 diabetes, gastrointestinal disease, kidney failure, genetic disorders and alcohol dependence. Deficiency can cause inflammation in the body, which is a common factor in many chronic diseases. This essential mineral also helps to protect our cells against oxidative stress, and deficiency can adversely affect our endothelial cells, which are a type of cell that forms a single layer lining the inside of blood vessels and lymphatic vessels, which are vital for transporting our immune cells and play a role in the body's defence against infections and diseases. Ultimately, a deficiency in magnesium may lead to endothelial dysfunction and increased inflammation as well as promote the development of numerous chronic diseases, including atherosclerosis, hypertension (high blood pressure) and coronary artery disease.

Magnesium-rich foods include beans, pulses, nuts, seeds, leafy green vegetables, avocado and dark chocolate. Despite these common food sources of magnesium, deficiency is common. Therefore, whether to supplement with magnesium depends on if you have a deficiency, and your own individual requirements. It can be useful to discuss potential supplementation with a dietician or nutritionist.

Other Immunity-Nourishing Nutrients

OMEGA-3S

Omega-3 polyunsaturated fats are essential to health. They reduce inflammation, prevent damage to our body's tissues and are beneficial to health. Our body is unable to make these fatty acids, so we need to get them through our diet.

The best food sources of omega-3 are oily fish, such as salmon, mackerel and sardines. However, some people don't like fish or don't manage to eat two servings a week, so omega-3 supplementation can be a good idea in these cases.

> Clinical signs of **omega-3 deficiency** include:
> - a rash that may be dry and scaly in appearance
> - increased risk of infections
> - poor wound healing
> - fertility issues
> - hair loss
> - reduced growth in children.

When choosing an omega-3 supplement, look for a combination of eicosapentaenoic acid (EPA) and docosahexaenoic acid (DHA). A third type of omega-3 is alpha-linolenic acid (ALA), which is a plant source, but unfortunately this is poorly converted to EPA and DHA.

Research has shown that omega-3 supplements can help reduce pain in joints in rheumatoid arthritis, and improve symptoms in inflammatory bowel disease and psoriasis. Recent studies have also shown that omega-3 fatty acids can cross into the brain and could help to reduce inflammation, which has been reported to play a role in Alzheimer's disease. Both human and animal studies have confirmed the ability of omega-3 fatty acids to impact the gut–brain axis, acting through gut microbiota composition. Our gut microbiome also plays an important part in helping us benefit from omega-3 fatty acids.

Currently, there are no official guidelines as to how much omega-3 we should be consuming per day or supplementing with. So, if you can eat fatty fish, aim to include two servings a week, and if you are unable to eat fish, consider introducing omega-3 supplements or algae supplements, which provide both DHA and EPA, if preferred.

PROBIOTICS

Probiotics are live microorganisms that provide benefits to gut health, which in turn helps to support the immune system. Probiotic live bacteria are found naturally in fermented foods but can also be taken as supplementation. Currently, we don't have enough evidence to determine which probiotic a healthy person should take to guarantee a beneficial and positive result. However, some specific probiotics have been confirmed to provide benefits for certain health issues. For example, if you have a sensitive stomach, the British Dietetic Association advise taking probiotics for a minimum of four weeks.

Choosing a probiotic supplement can be a minefield as some have a number of different strains, but probiotics are strain- and population-specific. This means that probiotic bacteria of the same genus and species can possess different functions depending on their strain. It can be very useful to discuss exactly which probiotic may help you most with a gut-health specialist.

My advice, if you are keen to supplement with a probiotic, is to choose one that has been proven to benefit gut health and immune function. A well-studied probiotic known as *Saccharomyces boulardii* is a type of yeast which modulates our gastrointestinal immune system and has been shown to provide gut-immune support. In addition to its anti-inflammatory abilities during infections, *Saccharomyces boulardii* can also support the host immune system by encouraging the release of immunoglobulins (a class of proteins that act as antibodies) and cytokines (a category of small proteins important in cell signalling).

Additionally, gold-standard, randomized controlled trials have shown that specific strains of *Bifidobacteria* and *Lactobacilli* supplements could also be effective in supporting immune function. These bacteria have immunomodulatory properties and have been reported to be beneficial in preventing and treating various infections, allergies and inflammatory conditions. The exact mechanisms are still being researched, but studies indicate that these probiotics can impact immune cell activity, modulate cytokine production and improve gut barrier function.

> Generally, **probiotics** are not required to be kept in the fridge as they return to their active state once in the gut.

If you are keen to follow a food-first approach and wish to save yourself money, focus on including a wide variety of fermented foods in your diet, such as live natural yoghurt, miso, kimchi and sauerkraut.

MYCONUTRIENTS

The key role of functional mushrooms in modulating immune function is a perfect example of how traditional practices can impact modern-day health. These powerful, medicinal mushrooms can be found in numerous different forms, such as tea, coffee, tincture and supplements.

Some of the most evidence-based mushrooms include:

Lion's mane (Hericium erinaceus)

This is a type of nootropic, which means that it contains unique myconutrients which may provide several brain health benefits. Research indicates that this is because of compounds such as hericenones and erinacines that promote the release of nerve growth factor (NGF) and brain-derived neurotrophic factor (BDNF). NGF and BDNF are both essential for the growth and protection of brain cells and increased cognitive function. Studies have also suggested that lion's mane can promote the innate immune response and promote intestinal immune function, providing a positive effect on both brain and immune health. Most individuals can supplement safely with 500–1,000mg daily; however, always consult with your doctor before supplementing with lion's mane or any other mushrooms, in case they interact with any medications that you are taking.

Chaga (Inonotus obliquus)

This medicinal mushroom is very rich in health-promoting antioxidants and contains a high amount of melanin, which gives Chaga its black colouring. It has been used for therapeutic purposes since the 16th century. Collections of folk medicine record Chaga being used to treat gastrointestinal cancer, diabetes, bacterial infection and liver diseases.

Modern research provides scientific evidence of the therapeutic effects of Chaga extracts, such as anti-inflammatory, antioxidant, anticancer, anti-diabetic, anti-obesity, anti-fatigue, antibacterial and antiviral activities.[1]

It is also heralded for its ability to support the immune system. These potent antioxidants decrease inflammation and promote immune health.

Reishi (Ganoderma lucidum)
Reishi is a mushroom that has been used in Eastern medicine for thousands of years and has been described as the 'mushroom of immortality'. It is known for its adaptogenic effects, meaning it helps the body to manage stress. Research indicates that this mushroom may protect us against stress-associated damage as well as aid us to manage stress-induced anxiety. It is also reported to support the adrenal gland, which plays an important role in the body's stress response by releasing cortisol.

Reishi contains triterpene, which has powerful immune-modulating and anti-inflammatory properties. It also provides the mushroom with a bitterness which is quite earthy and can be a fairly intense flavour, which does take some time getting used to if you aren't a fan of bitter tastes.

Cordyceps
This is another mushroom that can potentially help immune function, with one study confirming its potential benefit in participants who supplemented with 1.7g of cordyceps mycelium culture extract.[2] The researchers reported that this supplementation with cordyceps resulted in a 38 per cent increase in the activity of natural killer (NK) cells, our essential white blood cells that protect against infection.

COLLAGEN

If you are struggling to sleep, which can have a huge impact on your immunity as well as on your gut health and overall health, then research suggests that supplementing with 3g of glycine a day may be beneficial. Glycine is the main amino acid in collagen, the main structural protein of connective tissue, such as bone, skin, ligaments, tendons and cartilage.

You can promote glycine intake by supplementing with collagen, which may be more effective, as glycine competes with other amino acids for absorption and is potentially absorbed less efficiently by itself than when it's bound to other amino acids. However, I always recommend a diet-first approach, so focus on consuming a balanced diet that is rich in protein as a primary source of collagen and other essential nutrients.

Supplementation For Some

As we saw earlier, in times of stress our immune health can be severely threatened, and during this time supplementation may be useful, especially if appetite is suppressed and you are finding it difficult to eat. Stress can play a major role in nutritional deficiencies and can lead to a suppressed immune system as well as poorer gut health, insufficient sleep and a lower quality of life. Therefore, supplementing may be useful if you are undergoing a period of intense stress.

Chronically Stressed?

High levels of stress increase vitamin C requirements, so if you are experiencing extreme stress, you may be at an increased risk of deficiency. Research has shown that in individuals who are chronically stressed, supplementing with vitamin C at the start of a cold decreased the severity of symptoms.

Older Adult?

An older adult may benefit from supplementing as nutrient absorption is not as effective as we get older and also nutritional requirements increase during this time.

One supplement I do advise for anyone over 60 years old is vitamin B12. This is because as we age it is harder for us to absorb this vitamin.

If you are older or under significant stress, then a multivitamin supplement could be helpful. One randomized control study confirmed that elderly people who took a multivitamin had decreased risk of infections, experienced half the number of infections and improved immunity significantly.[3]

Strict Vegan Diet?

If you follow a strict vegan diet, then you may find yourself low in certain nutrients, including vitamin D, vitamin B12, iodine and omega-3 fatty acids, and supplementation may be helpful to ensure you are meeting requirements and to prevent a nutritional deficiency.

Pregnant?

During pregnancy, certain supplements may help support both mum and baby, such as supplementing with 400mcg of vitamin B9 (folic acid) until you are 12 weeks pregnant, as per NHS recommendations. This is to reduce the risk of problems in the baby's development in the early weeks of pregnancy.

The NHS also recommends pregnant women take a daily vitamin D supplement. However, do not supplement with cod liver oil or any vitamin A supplements when pregnant as too much vitamin A could potentially cause harm to your baby. It is very important to check supplement labels to confirm you are not taking toxic doses of any nutrient, especially when pregnant.

Perimenopausal?

Perimenopausal women may also benefit from certain nutritional supplementations to help manage some symptoms, including vitamin D to support bone health as it helps your body to absorb and use calcium. Our bone strength starts to decrease in our perimenopause years, so we need to do all we can to protect our bones. This is because oestrogen, which helps our bones to stay strong, decreases during this time.

As we have seen, vitamin D also plays a vital role in our immune health, and our immune function can also decrease during the perimenopause years. Therefore, you may wish to supplement with vitamin D, especially during the winter months or if you have diagnosed low levels.

> **Drug–nutrient interaction** is a very important consideration that is not discussed enough. Many people are taking supplements alongside medications, and these are interacting adversely with some dangerous implications.
>
> Always check with your medical practitioner before taking supplementation if you are on any other medication.

Summary

For most healthy individuals, I recommend focusing on your diet to meet your daily vitamin and mineral requirements as every food is made up of differing amounts of macronutrients (carbohydrates, proteins and fats), micronutrients (vitamins and minerals), fibre and other important nutrients such as phytonutrients (plant compounds). In the case of vitamin D, which is mainly synthesized through exposing our skin to the sun's UV rays, it is a slightly different recommendation, and you may find you need to supplement, especially if you have been diagnosed with suboptimal levels.

However, we do know that too much of something is not always a good thing when it comes to micronutrient supplementation, and this can result in potentially significant adverse side effects. Research has found that supplementing with high doses of vitamins A, B9 (folic acid), C, D and E may damage health, so when supplementing, ensure you keep to the recommended level of that particular nutrient.

To make an informed decision about dietary supplement use, I would advise that you speak with a dietician or nutritionist who can explain their benefits and risks and if supplementation is appropriate for you.

CHAPTER 12

The Immunity Plan – Putting It All Together

This table summarizes all the advice and recommendations that are included in *The Immunity Plan* in a way which I hope is easy for you to follow.

Please note that the stipulated recommendations in the below table are based on the UK government daily dietary guidelines for adults aged 18–64.

	DAILY RECOMMENDATION	FOODS
Total Energy	2,000 kcal (women) 2,500 kcal (men)	
Carbohydrates	267g (women) 333g (men)	Whole grains, legumes (beans, lentils, chickpeas) and starchy vegetables (butternut squash, swede, potatoes).
Fat (Total)	78g (women) 97g (men)	Salmon, mackerel, sardines, trout, olive oil, avocado, nuts and seeds.
Saturated Fat	24g (women) 31g (men)	
Protein	45g (women) 56g (men)	Eggs, fish, shellfish, chicken, turkey, beef, dairy products, chickpeas, beans, lentils, nuts and seeds.
Fibre	30g (women/men)	Whole grains, legumes (beans, lentils, chickpeas), vegetables and fruits.

Added/Free Sugars	30g (women/men) This is roughly equivalent to 7 sugar cubes.	Any sugars added to food or drinks (biscuits, chocolate, fizzy drinks) or sugars in honey, maple syrup, unsweetened fruit juices and smoothies.
Salt	6g (women/men) This is around 1 teaspoon.	Natural sources, such as seafood, meat and eggs.
Vitamin A	0.6mg (women) 0.7mg (men)	Liver (avoid if pregnant), cheese, eggs, milk, yoghurt, leafy dark green vegetables (kale, spinach) and orange vegetables (sweet potatoes, carrots, butternut squash).
Vitamin D	10mcg (women/men)	Oily fish (salmon, sardines mackerel), red meat, egg yolks, fortified foods (cereals, spreads), liver (avoid if pregnant) and mushrooms.
Vitamin E	3mg (women) 4mg (men)	Plant oils (rapeseed, sunflower, olive), nuts, seeds and wheatgerm (found in cereals).
Vitamin K	1mcg per kg of body weight (women/men) – e.g. for someone weighing 60kg this would be 60mcg	Leafy green vegetables (broccoli, spinach, kale), cereal grains and vegetable oils. *Small amounts can be found in meat and dairy products.*
Vitamin B6	1.2mg (women) 1.4mg (men)	Chicken, turkey, peanuts, wheatgerm, oats, bananas, milk and some fortified breakfast cereals.
Vitamin B9	200mcg (women/men)	Broccoli, Brussels sprouts, leafy green vegetables (kale, spring greens, spinach), chickpeas, kidney beans and liver (avoid if pregnant).
Vitamin B12	1.5mcg (women/men)	Meat, fish, milk, cheese, eggs and some fortified breakfast cereals.
Vitamin C	40mg (women/men)	Oranges, peppers, strawberries, broccoli, kiwi and tomatoes.
Copper	1.2mg (women/men)	Offal, shellfish and nuts.

Iron	14.8mg (women aged 19–49) 8.7mg (women aged 50+) 8.7mg (men)	Liver (avoid if pregnant), red meat, kidney beans, edamame beans, chickpeas, nuts, dried fruit and fortified breakfast cereals.
Magnesium	270mg (women) 300mg (men)	Wholemeal bread, spinach and nuts.
Selenium	60mcg (women) 75mcg (men)	Brazil nuts, cashews, sunflower seeds, eggs, chicken, fish and shellfish.
Zinc	7mg (women) 9.5mg (men)	Meat, shellfish, dairy foods, bread, whole-grain cereal products, pine nuts and pumpkin seeds.
Omega-3	2 portions of fish per week – including 1 serving of oily fish (women/men). 1 portion is approximately 140mg (cooked). *Oily fish have higher levels of pollutants; therefore, the following individuals should eat no more than 2 portions of oily fish a week – girls, women who are planning a pregnancy, women who are pregnant or breastfeeding.*	Oily fish (salmon, sardines, mackerel, trout, kipper, pilchards, sprats) and white fish (cod, haddock, plaice, pollock, tilapia).
Probiotics	No defined guideline – I recommend including 2 servings per day.	Fermented foods, such as natural live yoghurt (no added sugar), sauerkraut, kimchi, kefir, kombucha and miso.
Prebiotics	No defined guideline – I recommend including several different food sources per day.	Apples, bananas, apricots, onions, garlic, leeks, almonds, cashews, wheat, rye, spelt, chickpeas, black beans, silken tofu, lentils and soya.

	RECOMMENDATION	
Physical Activity	150 minutes moderate-intensity activity per week.	Brisk walking, bike riding, doubles tennis, pushing a lawn mower, hiking and dancing.
	OR	
	75 minutes vigorous-intensity activity per week.	Running, fast swimming, HIIT, riding a bike fast or uphill, football, netball, hocket, skipping and martial arts.
	AND	
	2 strengthening/weight-bearing sessions per week that work all muscle groups.	Pilates, yoga, weight training, tai chi, body weight exercises (squats, lunges, push-ups) and heavy gardening (digging, shovelling). Even carrying heavy shopping bags or lifting and carrying children counts!
Sunlight	Aim to get 10–15 minutes of sun exposure several times per week.	Expose your face, arms and legs, if possible. *However, balance is vital, and if you are out in the sun for long periods, please do protect or cover up skin to reduce the risk of skin damage and skin cancer.*
Sleep	Aim to get 7–9 hours of sleep per night.	Ensure you relax and wind down before bed to prevent sleep issues.

PART 3

The Recipes

These recipes are suitable for after you have completed The Good Gut Health Plan.

Breakfast

Mixed Berry Porridge

Oats are an excellent source of both soluble and insoluble fibre, which are essential for gut health as well as healthy digestion. Oats are also rich in beta-glucan, a type of soluble fibre that acts as a prebiotic, meaning it nourishes beneficial bacteria in the gut, promoting a balanced gut microbiome. This important prebiotic fibre 'feeds' our beneficial gut bacteria so they can carry out their important roles, including supporting our immune system.

This recipe is loaded with antioxidant-rich berries that help to fight harmful free radicals, protecting our body's cells from damage that could lead to illness and disease. The natural Greek yoghurt is an excellent source of probiotics (live bacteria) that help boost our gut health and keep the beneficial bacteria topped up!

SERVES 2

- 80g porridge oats
- ½ tsp ground cinnamon
- 150ml milk of choice
- 1 small egg
- 2 tbsp maple syrup (optional)
- 100g strawberries
- 100g raspberries
- 100g blueberries
- 2 tbsp natural Greek yoghurt

1. Preheat the oven to 180°C/160°C fan/gas mark 4.
2. Add the oats and cinnamon to a large bowl.
3. Add the milk, egg and maple syrup (optional) to a jug and whisk well.
4. In a second bowl, add the berries and mix together.
5. In a baking dish, add half of the berries, then top with the oats and cinnamon mixture.
6. Pour in the milk, egg and maple syrup mixture and scatter the remaining half of the berries over.
7. Place in the oven and cook for 25 minutes.
7. Serve with Greek yoghurt.

Pecan Protein Pancakes

Pecans are beneficial for both gut health and the immune system due to their fibre content and the presence of numerous vitamins and minerals, including magnesium, which has anti-inflammatory benefits and can help reduce inflammation throughout the body and potentially improve immune responses. Additionally, pecans contain antioxidants like vitamin E and zinc, which support immune cell development and function, helping the body fight infections.

This recipe also contains banana, which is rich in prebiotic fibre. This fuels our beneficial gut bacteria and helps to produce short-chain fatty acids that are crucial for immune and gut health. Bananas also provide essential nutrients like vitamin C, vitamin B6 and potassium, which support overall immune function.

When bananas are unripe or green, they are particularly high in resistant starch; however, as they ripen the resistant starch decreases while the sugar content increases. In this recipe, I would suggest using ripe bananas as they are easier to mash, but try and also include unripe bananas in your diet as a snack.

THE IMMUNITY PLAN

SERVES 2

- 2 bananas, mashed
- 1 egg
- ¼ tsp baking powder
- 1 tbsp peanut butter powder
- 2 tsp extra virgin olive oil
- 60g pecans, chopped
- 100g natural Greek yoghurt

1. Add the mashed bananas into a bowl.

2. Whisk the eggs in a small jug or bowl.

3. Add the eggs to the banana with the baking powder and peanut butter powder and whisk until smooth.

4. Over a medium heat, add the olive oil to a pan. For each individual pancake add 2 spoonfuls of the pancake mixture.

5. Cook for 2 minutes then flip and cook the other side for 2 minutes. Once firm and cooked through, transfer to a large plate and cook the next pancake. Repeat until all the mixture is used.

6. Sprinkle over the chopped pecans and serve with Greek yoghurt.

Overnight Fruit and Nut Oats

Oats contain a higher protein content compared to many other widely consumed cereals, such as corn and rice. They also have a fairly good balance of essential amino acids. Additionally, oats have antioxidant and anti-inflammatory properties, and according to the Food and Drug Administration and European Food Safety Authority nutrient source guidance, they are a good source of protein, fibre, iron, magnesium, phosphorus, zinc, copper, manganese and selenium.

This recipe contains walnuts, which are rich in health-promoting plant compounds (polyphenols) that have antioxidant effects, helping to protect our cells from damage. A specific type of polyphenol found in walnuts, ellagitannins, may be particularly beneficial. These compounds can be converted by gut bacteria into urolithins, which have anti-inflammatory properties and may protect against inflammation.

THE IMMUNITY PLAN

SERVES 2

- 80g oats
- 150g natural Greek yoghurt
- 150ml milk of choice
- 2 tsp maple syrup (optional)
- 5 dried apricots
- 200g fresh or frozen mixed berries
- 8 walnut halves
- 2 tsp cacao nibs (optional)

1. In a large mixing bowl, add the oats, Greek yoghurt, milk, maple syrup (optional) and apricots.

2. Top with the berries and walnuts. Cover the bowl and put into the fridge for 12 hours or overnight.

3. Remove from the fridge, spoon into two bowls and scatter over the cacao nibs (optional).

Raspberry and Almond Pot

Greek yoghurt is protein-rich and high in many other nutrients like vitamin B12, calcium and the immune-supporting mineral selenium. Almonds are the edible seeds of Prunus dulcis, *more commonly called the almond tree. They are rich in vitamin E, which is a powerful antioxidant that is key to a healthy immune system. Vitamin E is a fat-soluble vitamin, which means it requires the presence of fat to be absorbed properly. Almonds are also rich in minerals such as manganese and magnesium which play an important role in promoting mood as well as sleep.*

Not only are raspberries delicious, but they are high in several powerful antioxidant compounds, including vitamin C, quercetin and ellagic acid that help to support immune function.

SERVES 2
- 250g natural Greek yoghurt
- 100g frozen raspberries
- 4 tsp roasted almonds, chopped

1. Add the Greek yoghurt and frozen raspberries to a food processor and pulse to break up the fruit and mix into the yoghurt.

2. Separate into two bowls and sprinkle over the chopped almonds.

Sliced Nutty Apple

Apples support our immune system and gut health as they are packed with prebiotic fibre and polyphenols (powerful plant compounds) which nourish beneficial gut bacteria and promote a diverse, balanced gut microbiome.

Flaxseeds are also an excellent source of prebiotic fibre, which 'feeds' our beneficial gut bacteria so they can carry out their vital roles. They also contain insoluble fibre, which promotes bowel regularity. Flaxseeds are a good source of omega-3 fatty acids as well as beneficial plant compounds like lignans.

Hazelnuts are a rich source of vitamins and minerals like vitamin E, manganese and copper. Additionally, they have a high content of omega-3 fatty acids.

THE IMMUNITY PLAN

SERVES 2

- 1 large apple, pips removed and cut into 4 round slices
- 2 tbsp cream cheese
- 2 tbsp frozen berries, defrosted
- 2 tbsp ground flaxseeds
- 80g hazelnuts, chopped

1. Place the 4 round apple slices on a plate and spread them with the cream cheese.
2. Add the berries on top of the cream cheese and sprinkle with the flaxseeds and hazelnuts.

Lunch

Brunch Bruschetta

Eggs are a complete protein source, meaning they contain all nine essential amino acids that the body needs to build and repair tissues, including immune cells and antibodies. They are also rich in various nutrients that play vital roles in immune function, such as vitamins A, B12, D and E, as well as the minerals selenium and zinc and antioxidants like lutein and zeaxanthin.

Whole-grain and dark rye breads are less processed than white breads and tend to have more nutrients. Research shows that eating whole grains is beneficial for overall health as they contain significant amounts of fibre, vitamins and minerals, such as iron and zinc. The fibre in whole-grain or rye bread can also help you feel fuller for longer.

THE IMMUNITY PLAN

SERVES 2

- 1 tsp extra virgin olive oil
- ½ red onion, finely chopped
- 1 yellow pepper, deseeded and thinly sliced
- 1 carrot, grated
- 1 garlic clove, crushed
- 3 large eggs
- 2 x 50g toasted whole-grain or rye bread slices
- Freshly ground black pepper

1. Over a medium heat, add the olive oil to a pan and cook the onion, pepper, carrot and garlic for 5 minutes, until softened.

2. Beat the eggs then add them to the pan. Stir and cook for 2–3 minutes or until the eggs are firm.

3. Place the eggs on top of the toast and season with the black pepper.

Stuffed Portobello Mushrooms

Portobello mushrooms offer several benefits for our immune health due to their rich nutrient profile. They contain selenium, vitamin D and vitamin B6, all of which are vital for immune function. The antioxidants and phytonutrients present in these mushrooms also contribute to overall immune support.

Additionally, portobello mushrooms contain beta-glucans (a type of prebiotic fibre), which can reduce inflammation, support gut health and modulate the immune system. Beta-glucans can also help to promote the growth of certain beneficial bacteria, such as **Bifidobacteria** *and* **Lactobacilli***.*

Portobellos contain antioxidants, such as the 'master' antioxidant, glutathione, and ergothioneine, which help protect cells from damage and support immune function. These mushrooms also contain compounds such as L-ergothioneine and conjugated linoleic acid, which have been shown to have anticancer properties and may also contribute to immune system health.

SERVES 4

- 8 large portobello mushrooms, stalks removed
- 2 tsp olive oil
- 2 red onions, roughly chopped
- 4 garlic cloves, finely chopped
- 2 tsp smoked paprika
- 2 yellow peppers, roughly chopped
- 2 large tomatoes, chopped
- 4 red chillies, deseeded and finely chopped
- 150g spinach
- 80g Cheddar cheese, grated
- Freshly ground black pepper

1. Preheat the oven to 220°C/200°C fan/gas mark 7.
2. Place the mushrooms, skin-side down, on to a roasting tin and set aside.
3. Add the olive oil to a large pan, and over a medium heat, add the red onions and fry for 2 minutes until softened.
4. Add the garlic, paprika and peppers, stir well and cook for 2 minutes.
5. Add in the tomatoes and red chillies and cook for a further 2–3 minutes.
6. Add the spinach and 1–2 tbsp water, if needed, and stir-fry for 2 minutes or until the spinach is wilted.
7. Mix in half of the cheese and stir well.
8. Remove the mixture from the heat and spoon it into the mushrooms, dividing the mixture equally.
9. Sprinkle over the rest of the cheese and place the roasting tin in the oven on the middle shelf for 15–20 minutes.
10. Season to taste with freshly ground pepper, and serve with a green salad dressed with homemade vinaigrette.

Zesty Spinach Soup

Spinach is a good source of vitamin C, a powerful antioxidant that plays a crucial role in immune function. It helps protect cells from damage and supports the production of white blood cells, which are essential for fighting off infections. Spinach also contains beta-carotene, an antioxidant that is converted into vitamin A in the body and helps antibodies respond to toxins and viruses. This leafy green vegetable is a great source of vitamin E, iron, potassium and magnesium.

Tahini, a paste made from ground sesame seeds, offers several health benefits due to its rich nutrient profile. It is packed with essential nutrients, including calcium, iron, magnesium, phosphorus and selenium. It's also a good source of B vitamins, vitamin E and healthy fats. Tahini also contains antioxidants and anti-inflammatory compounds, with studies suggesting it may contribute to improved heart health and reduced inflammation, and it potentially even exerts a cancer-fighting effect.

THE IMMUNITY PLAN

SERVES 4

- 2 tbsp extra virgin olive oil
- 1 large white onion, chopped
- 1.5l vegetable stock, low salt
- 450g baby spinach
- 2 tbsp tahini
- 1 tbsp lemon zest

1. Over a medium heat, add the olive oil to a large saucepan and add the onion. Cook for 5 minutes until softened.

2. Add the vegetable stock, bring to the boil and simmer for 5 minutes.

3. Add the baby spinach and cook for a further 2–3 minutes.

4. Add the tahini and lemon zest and stir. Cook for 1 minute.

5. Transfer the soup to a blender and blend until smooth.

Green Lentil Soup

Lentils are edible seeds of the legume family and come in a variety of colours including red, green, brown, yellow and black. They are a rich source of nutrition, providing plenty of protein, fibre and numerous essential micronutrients. In fact, as much as a third of the calories from lentils comes from protein. Similar to other legumes, lentils are low in a couple of the essential amino acids, namely methionine and cysteine; however, this is easily addressed by combining lentils with cereal grains, such as rice or wheat, so just add a couple of slices of whole-grain bread to accompany this delicious lentil soup.

In addition, lentils can have a powerful antioxidant, anti-inflammatory, antiviral and antibacterial effect. Research indicates that eating lentils on a regular basis can reduce your risk of chronic disease, such as diabetes, obesity, cancer and heart disease. This is believed to be due to the protective plant compounds called phenols that are abundant in lentils.

SERVES 4

- 200g dried green lentils
- 1 tbsp extra virgin olive oil
- 1 white onion, finely chopped
- 2 garlic cloves, finely chopped
- 1 celery stick, chopped
- 1.5l vegetable stock, low salt
- 400g tin chopped tomatoes
- 1 carrot, sliced
- 1 tsp dried oregano
- 120g kale, stalks removed, chopped
- Freshly ground pepper

1. Soak the lentils in cold water overnight or for at least 12 hours.

2. Drain the lentils and rinse well.

3. Over a medium heat, add the olive oil to a large saucepan or casserole dish. Add the onion, garlic and celery and cook for 5 minutes, until softened.

4. Add the stock, tomatoes, carrot and oregano and bring to the boil. Add the lentils and reduce the heat to low. Simmer for 30–35 minutes, stirring every few minutes. Cook until the lentils are tender.

5. Add the kale and simmer for a further 15 minutes.

6. Season with freshly ground pepper and serve with whole-grain or rye bread.

Fabulous Frittata

Eggs are one of the best dietary sources of an essential nutrient called choline, which is vital for the formation of our cell membranes and memory. Choline is also key for liver health as it helps transport fat out of the liver, and when a person is deficient in choline, this can increase the risk of getting a fatty liver, which can lead to significant health issues. Being deficient in choline can affect the expression of genes involved in the process of our cells multiplying. During the development of a foetus, choline deficiency can be particularly harmful because it inhibits cell proliferation in the brain.

One study involving almost 1,400 individuals aged 36–83 demonstrated that those with a higher choline intake tended to have better memories, and that choline intake during midlife may help to protect our brains.

In this frittata, I use goat's cheese as it is a good source of probiotics, beneficial bacteria that support our gut health and digestion. Also, many people find goat's cheese easier to digest than cheese made from cow's milk due to its lower lactose content and different protein structure.

THE IMMUNITY PLAN

SERVES 4

- 150g frozen peas
- 200g asparagus spears, ends trimmed, cut into approx. 5cm lengths
- 5 large eggs
- 120g Parmesan, grated
- 2 tbsp extra virgin olive oil
- 100g goat's cheese, chopped

1. In a large pan, add water and bring to the boil. Add the frozen peas and bring back to the boil.

2. Add the asparagus and cook for 4 minutes until tender.

3. Drain the vegetables and set aside.

4. While the vegetables are boiling, whisk the eggs in a large bowl.

5. Add the grated Parmesan, peas and asparagus and mix.

6. Heat the grill to a high temperature and heat a frying pan over a medium heat.

7. Add the olive oil to the frying pan and carefully pour in the egg mixture. Make sure the asparagus and peas are spread out evenly. Cook for 4 minutes.

8. Scatter over the chopped goat's cheese and place under the grill for 4 minutes until golden brown.

Asparagus and Mozzarella Salad

Asparagus provides essential vitamins like A, C and E, which are known for their antioxidant properties and role in immune cell function. It also contains folate, a B vitamin crucial for immune cell production and overall immune health. This tasty vegetable is packed with the 'master' antioxidant glutathione, which helps neutralize harmful free radicals in the body and reduce oxidative stress and inflammation, which are linked to various diseases and can suppress immunity.

In addition, asparagus contains inulin, a type of fibre that acts as a prebiotic, promoting the growth of beneficial gut bacteria. It also contains compounds such as polyphenols that have anti-inflammatory effects. Chronic inflammation can suppress the immune system, so reducing inflammation can indirectly support immune function.

Mozzarella cheese can offer benefits for gut and immune health due to its probiotic content. These probiotics, like **Lactobacillus casei** *and* **Lactobacillus fermentum,** *may improve digestion and potentially reduce inflammation, while also contributing to a healthy immune response. As well as being a good protein source, mozzarella provides essential vitamins and minerals like calcium, phosphorus and immune-nourishing zinc.*

SERVES 4

- 350g cherry tomatoes, halved
- 2 tbsp extra virgin olive oil
- 2 garlic cloves, finely chopped
- 500g asparagus, trimmed
- 1 tbsp balsamic vinegar
- 150g mozzarella, torn into pieces
- Freshly ground black pepper

1. Preheat the oven to 200°C/180°C fan/gas mark 6.
2. Add the cherry tomatoes to a dish and drizzle with 1 tbsp of the olive oil.
3. Stir the garlic into the tomatoes. Place in the oven and cook for 8–10 minutes.
4. Place the asparagus on a baking tray and drizzle with the remaining 1 tbsp of olive oil.
5. Remove the cherry tomatoes from the oven and stir in the balsamic vinegar.
6. Put the tomatoes back in the oven on the bottom shelf and the asparagus on the top shelf. Cook for 10 minutes, stirring the asparagus halfway through cooking.
7. Remove the asparagus from the oven and arrange in a large serving dish with the mozzarella.
8. Remove the tomatoes from the oven and place over the asparagus and mozzarella.
9. Season with freshly ground black pepper.

Wild Rice Salad

Wild rice, a whole grain that has been growing in popularity in recent years, is a good source of protein, manganese, phosphorus and magnesium. It is also a source of zinc, a mineral that supports the development and activity of immune cells, helping the body fight off infection. Wild rice contains resistant starch, which acts as a prebiotic, nourishing our beneficial gut bacteria and helping to maintain a balanced and diverse gut microbiome.

In this recipe, I also use apple cider vinegar, which is believed to offer several benefits for immune health, primarily due to its antimicrobial properties and potential impact on gut health. The acetic acid in apple cider vinegar can help fight harmful bacteria and viruses while the probiotics it contains can support a healthy gut microbiome, which plays a crucial role in immune function.

SERVES 4

- 150g wild rice
- 2 tbsp extra virgin olive oil
- 1 red onion, finely chopped
- 3 tsp natural Greek yoghurt
- 2 tsp lemon juice
- 2 tsp apple cider vinegar
- 4 dates, pitted and thinly sliced
- 2 celery sticks, chopped
- 50g flaked almonds, toasted
- Freshly ground black pepper

1. Cook the rice as per pack instructions and set aside to cool.

2. Add 1 tbsp of the olive oil to a pan, and over a medium heat, cook the onion for 5 minutes.

3. Meanwhile, add the remaining 1 tbsp of olive oil, the Greek yoghurt, lemon juice and apple cider vinegar to a bowl and whisk together.

4. In a separate large bowl, add the cooled rice, onion, dates, celery and almonds, and stir. Add the yoghurt dressing and mix.

5. Season with freshly ground black pepper.

Miso Aubergines

Miso, a fermented soybean paste, is a super fermented food source. It is rich in live bacteria that can benefit our gut health and promote a healthy gut microbiome, which plays a crucial role in immune function. Additionally, miso contains various vitamins and minerals, including manganese and zinc, which are important for immune cell function and overall immune health. Miso's isoflavone content has been linked to a reduced risk of certain cancers, including stomach and breast cancer.

Aubergines are one of my favourite vegetables and contain vitamins A, C and E, which are essential for immune function and overall health. They are also a good source of vitamin B6, which is important for the proper functioning of immune cells and helps the body fight off infections. The purple skin of aubergines is packed with anthocyanins, powerful antioxidants that protect cells from damage caused by harmful free radicals. Also, some compounds in aubergines, like chlorogenic acid, have anti-inflammatory properties that can indirectly benefit the immune system. Research indicates that another compound, solasodine rhamnosyl glycosides, may have cancer-fighting properties, potentially supporting the immune system's ability to recognize and eliminate cancerous cells.

THE IMMUNITY PLAN

SERVES 4

- 1kg aubergines, cut in half lengthways
- Sprinkle of sea salt
- 3 tbsp miso
- 2 tbsp sake
- 1 tbsp soy sauce
- 1 tbsp honey
- Sprinkle of black and white sesame seeds

1. Take the aubergines and score the cut sides in a criss-cross pattern, making sure you don't cut too deep as you may lose the shape.

2. Sprinkle over the sea salt and leave for 8–10 minutes. Then rinse the aubergines, dry and wrap for a few minutes in kitchen paper.

3. Preheat the grill to a medium heat.

4. Place the aubergines on a baking try and cook under the grill for 12–15 minutes until they are cooked.

5. Meanwhile mix together the miso, sake, soy sauce and honey.

6. When the aubergines are completely cooked, remove from the grill and cover with the miso mixture. Sprinkle the sesame seeds over the aubergines.

7. Serve with whole-grain rice.

Ultimate Stir-Fry

A diverse gut microbiome, which is vital for immune health, thrives on a varied diet, including a wide range of plant-based foods. This ultimate stir-fry contains a large variety of plant foods in one meal, which is fantastic for ensuring a diverse diet. Recent research suggests that consuming 30 or more different plant-based foods per week can significantly benefit gut health. This theory emerged from research carried out as part of the American Gut Project, a crowd-sourced project involving more than 10,000 participants. They discovered that participants who ate 30 or more different types of plants per week had gut microbiomes that were the most diverse – and hence health-promoting.

This recipe includes shiitake mushrooms, which are known to provide numerous health benefits, including supporting immunity, due to their rich nutrient profile and bioactive compounds. Polysaccharides like lentinan, found in shiitake, can enhance immune function and help the body fight infection.

SERVES 4

- 1 tbsp extra virgin olive oil
- 1 red onion, finely sliced
- 1 carrot, sliced
- 1 red pepper, sliced
- 1 yellow pepper, sliced
- 120g shiitake mushrooms, sliced
- 2cm fresh root ginger, grated
- 1 garlic clove, finely chopped
- 1 red chilli, finely chopped
- 300g white cabbage, shredded
- 150g mangetout, trimmed
- ½ vegetable stock cube, low salt
- 500g courgette, spiralized or thinly sliced
- 2 tbsp lime juice

1. Over a high heat, add the olive oil to a large pan then add the onion, carrot, peppers and mushrooms, and cook for 5 minutes until softened.

2. Add the ginger, garlic and red chilli and cook for 1 minute.

3. Add the cabbage and mangetout, and cook for a further 2 minutes.

4. Meanwhile, dissolve half a stock cube in 3 tbsp of boiling water, then add the stock and courgette to the pan. Cook for 3 minutes until the vegetables are tender.

5. Add the lime juice and serve.

Tofu Butternut Burgers

Fermented tofu is rich in probiotics, the beneficial bacteria that contribute to a balanced gut microbiome. It also contains soy isoflavones, which can promote a healthy gut lining and reduce inflammation, potentially improving digestion and overall gut health. Tofu is an excellent source of plant protein, which is crucial for building and repairing tissues, including those involved in immune function, like antibodies. It also provides essential nutrients like iron and zinc, which are important for immune system function. Furthermore, tofu is a good source of calcium and magnesium, minerals essential for strong bones.

Butternut squash is a great source of beta-carotene, which the body converts to vitamin A, a micronutrient that is vital for immune function and helps the body fight off infections. It is also packed with fibre, promoting optimal digestion and gut health.

Nutritional yeast is a deactivated yeast with a savoury, cheese-like flavour that is often used as a vegan cheese substitute or seasoning. It's a good source of protein, B vitamins (including B12 in fortified products) and some minerals. It may also offer potential benefits such as supporting the immune system, lowering cholesterol and promoting gut health. Some yeast strains, such as **Saccharomyces cerevisiae**, *exert prebiotic effects that may promote a healthy gut microbiome.*

SERVES 4

- 400g firm tofu
- 300g butternut squash, peeled and grated
- 150g tahini
- 2 tbsp nutritional yeast
- 2 tbsp extra virgin olive oil
- Salad leaves
- 200g carrot, grated

1. Preheat the oven to 200°C/180°C fan/gas mark 6.
2. Press the tofu with kitchen paper to dry, then crumble it into a large bowl.
3. Add the grated butternut squash, tahini and nutritional yeast, and stir to combine.
4. Divide and form the mixture into 4 burger patties.
5. Over a medium heat, add the olive oil to a large frying pan and cook the patties for 4 minutes, then flip and cook the other side for 4 minutes.
6. Remove the patties from the pan and place on a baking sheet in the oven. Cook for 12 minutes.
7. Place the patties on the salad leaves and serve with the grated carrot.

Dinner

Creamy Vegetable Red Curry

This recipe is packed with a variety of plant foods and essential nutrients. In this curry, I use red and yellow peppers, which are rich in numerous vitamins and minerals, including vitamins A, C and K as well as B vitamins, such as B6 and folate (B9). Peppers are particularly high in vitamin C – in fact, one medium-sized red pepper provides approximately 170 per cent of the required daily intake of this immune-nourishing micronutrient.

Coconut milk is delicious, and it also has potential immune health benefits as it contains lauric acid, which the body converts to monolaurin, a compound with antimicrobial and antiviral properties. Monolaurin may help fight off harmful bacteria, viruses and fungi, thus providing immune system support. This plant-based milk is naturally lactose free and can be used as a milk substitute for individuals with lactose intolerance. Lactose is the main type of carbohydrate in all mammalian milk and is made up of two sugars. Your body needs an enzyme called lactase to adequately digest it, and it is this enzyme that is lacking in individuals with lactose intolerance.

THE IMMUNITY PLAN

SERVES 4

- 3 tbsp extra virgin olive oil
- 2 aubergines, quartered lengthways and cut into 2-inch pieces
- 1 onion, chopped
- 2 garlic cloves, finely chopped
- 4cm fresh ginger root, grated
- 3 tbsp red curry paste
- 400ml coconut milk
- 1 yellow pepper, sliced
- 1 red pepper, sliced
- 2 tbsp fish sauce
- 1 lime, ½ juiced and the other ½ cut into wedges

1. Preheat the oven to 220°C/200°C fan/gas mark 7.

2. Add the olive oil to a roasting tin and place in the oven for 3 minutes.

3. Add the aubergines, onion and garlic to the tin and stir. Place in the oven and cook for 18–20 minutes.

4. Add the ginger and red curry paste and stir, then cook for a further 5 minutes.

5. Add the coconut milk, yellow pepper, red pepper and fish sauce. Cook for a further 8 minutes.

6. Remove the tin from the oven and add the lime juice. Serve with the lime wedges and with whole-grain rice.

Turkey and Butternut Squash Lasagne

Turkey is low in fat and higher in protein than chicken, and the protein in turkey provides all nine essential amino acids that we need for growth and repair. It is high in selenium, zinc and B vitamins, all of which play a vital role in immune function. Selenium is a mineral that acts as an antioxidant and is essential for thyroid hormone metabolism, which in turn affects the immune system.

This recipe includes Parmesan cheese, which provides important probiotics, such as Lactobacillus *bacteria, which can help support a healthy gut microbiome, leading to improved digestion and nutrient absorption and a stronger, more balanced immune system. The fermentation process in Parmesan cheese produces health-promoting short-chain fatty acids and other compounds that can act as prebiotics, thereby nourishing our beneficial gut bacteria. Parmesan cheese is also a good source of protein and calcium and is notable for its easy digestibility.*

Lentils are also included in this recipe and are a good source of immune-supporting zinc, selenium, folate, copper, magnesium and manganese. Zinc is vital for the development of white blood cells and the synthesis of antibodies, both of which are essential for a healthy immune response. Lentils are also packed with protein and fibre, which support gut health. On top of this, they are a rich source of antioxidants, which can help protect our cells against damage, potentially reduce inflammation and support our immune system.

THE IMMUNITY PLAN

SERVES 4

- 1 butternut squash, peeled, deseeded and sliced
- 2 tbsp extra virgin olive oil
- 1 white onion, finely chopped
- 2 carrots, finely chopped
- 2 celery sticks, finely chopped
- 500g turkey mince
- 1 tbsp tomato puree
- 2 x 400g tins chopped tomatoes
- 120g dried lentils of any colour
- 350ml water
- 150g button mushrooms, sliced
- 80g Parmesan, finely grated

1. Preheat the oven to 200°C/180°C fan/gas mark 6.
2. Place the butternut squash slices on to a baking sheet and drizzle with 1 tbsp of the olive oil. Put into the oven for 18–20 minutes until the butternut squash is tender.
3. Meanwhile, over a medium heat, heat the remaining 1 tbsp of olive oil in a large pan.
4. Add the onion, carrots and celery, and cook for 4–5 minutes.
5. Turn up the heat to medium-high, add the mince and cook for 5–6 minutes. Stir frequently.
6. Add the tomato puree, chopped tomatoes, dried lentils and water, and bring to a simmer.
7. Cover with a lid and cook for 15 minutes.
8. Add the button mushrooms and cook for 12 minutes.

9. In a baking dish, transfer half the mince mixture and top with half of the butternut squash slices. Then transfer the remaining half of the mince and top with the remaining butternut squash slices.

10. Scatter over the Parmesan, place the baking dish into the oven and cook for 15 minutes.

Veggie Biryani

This biryani is made with whole-grain rice – I always use whole grains where possible as they can help with managing inflammation levels in the body. Diets which are high in fibre have been shown to reduce C-reactive protein levels, a key marker for inflammation, by up to 40 per cent. In addition, whole grains contain beta-glucans, a fibre that helps to promote immune health and decrease inflammation.

I use frozen peas in this recipe as they are cost effective and are a good source of immune-supporting nutrients like vitamins A, C and E as well as zinc and antioxidants that help protect us from infections. They also contain plant compounds like catechins, which support the immune system. Peas also contain prebiotics, which nourish the beneficial bacteria in the gut. While many people think fresh is always best, freezing peas can actually help preserve their nutritional value, particularly vitamin C, making them a convenient, affordable and nutritious option.

SERVES 4

- 350g whole-grain rice or brown basmati rice
- 750ml water
- 1 vegetable stock cube, low salt
- 3 tbsp curry paste (Madras or tikka work well)
- 1 tbsp olive oil
- 1 red pepper, sliced
- 1 yellow pepper, sliced
- 1 large onion, chopped
- 200g frozen peas
- 200g spinach, chopped
- 100g unsalted roasted cashew nuts, roughly chopped

1. Pour the rice into a large saucepan and add 750ml of cold water. Stir and crumble in the stock cube. Add the curry paste and bring to the boil.

2. Turn the heat down, stir, cover with a lid and cook for 20–22 minutes until all the water is absorbed and the rice is tender.

3. Turn the heat off and set aside for the rice to steam until the veggies have been prepared.

4. Add the olive oil to a pan over a medium heat then add the peppers, onion and frozen peas. Cook for 8 minutes, stirring well.

5. Add in the spinach and cook until it is wilted.

6. Once the vegetables are cooked, stir the vegetable mixture into the rice.

7. Divide between four serving bowls, sprinkle over the cashew nuts and serve.

Lemongrass Salmon

Salmon offers a wide array of health benefits, primarily due to its high content of omega-3 fatty acids, protein and various vitamins and minerals. These nutrients contribute to immune function, heart health and brain health and can even play a role in reducing inflammation and supporting healthy ageing. The omega-3s in salmon have anti-inflammatory effects, which may help with various conditions including arthritis and other inflammatory diseases.

Fatty fish, such as salmon, is often touted as brain food, and there's convincing evidence to support this. Research reports that regular consumption reduces age-related brain loss and may improve memory, due to the abundance of omega-3 fatty acids in the fish. Studies have confirmed beneficial effects on conditions such as the autoimmune disease multiple sclerosis as well as Alzheimer's disease and depression.

Traditionally, lemongrass has been used to aid digestion and may help with issues like bloating and indigestion. It is a good source of antioxidants and vitamins like A and C, which are important for immune function. Additionally, its antibacterial and antifungal properties may help fight off infections. Lemongrass also contains compounds such as citral and quercetin, which have anti-inflammatory effects and are reported to have anticancer properties. Quercetin is a flavonoid with powerful antioxidant properties. Lemongrass may help reduce inflammation and potentially alleviate symptoms of painful conditions like arthritis.

SERVES 4

- 4 tbsp light soy sauce
- 4 tbsp mirin
- 8 spring onions, thinly shredded
- 2 courgettes, halved and cut into thin sticks
- Freshly ground black pepper
- Sea salt
- 4 salmon fillets
- 4 lemongrass stalks, thinly shredded
- 30g fresh root ginger, grated
- 4 garlic cloves, thinly sliced

1. Preheat the oven to 200°C/180°C fan/gas mark 6.

2. In a bowl, mix the soy sauce and mirin.

3. Line a roasting tin with greaseproof paper. Add the spring onions and courgettes and season with salt and pepper.

4. Add the salmon on top of the vegetables, then add the lemongrass, ginger and garlic. Pour the soy sauce and mirin mixture over the salmon.

5. Fold the sides of the greaseproof paper over so they join in the middle and then fold the ends.

6. Place the roasting tin into the oven for 20 minutes until the fish flakes.

Stir-Fried Chinese Tofu

Tofu is a soy-based food that originated in China. It is made from soybeans, water and a class of ingredients called coagulants that keep the two together, and it comes in different varieties, categorized by firmness. It can be enjoyed in many ways, including baked, grilled, stir-fried and steamed. Tofu is rich in protein, calcium, manganese, copper and selenium, though the precise amount of nutrients, vitamins and minerals found in a given amount of tofu will vary by the brand and firmness you select.

This versatile plant protein can be beneficial for women experiencing perimenopausal symptoms due to its isoflavone (phytoestrogen that can mimic oestrogen in the body) content, which may help reduce hot flushes and potentially improve bone health. A soy-rich diet may also help reduce the risk of endometrial, colon, stomach and prostate cancers. One review of 13 studies found that high intakes of soy isoflavones were associated with a 19 per cent lower risk of endometrial cancer.

Tip – you can make your own tofu using whole soybeans, lemon juice and water.

SERVES 2

- 400g medium-firm tofu, drained
- 20g + 1 tbsp cornflour
- 2 eggs
- 3 tbsp extra virgin olive oil
- 2 spring onions, finely chopped
- 2 garlic cloves, finely chopped
- 200ml + 2 tbsp water
- 2 tbsp light soy sauce
- 1 tsp peanut or sesame oil

1. Cut the tofu into 1cm slices and dry with kitchen paper.

2. Put 20g of cornflour on a plate and coat each slice of tofu in the cornflour.

3. In a separate bowl, beat the eggs and place the tofu in the eggs.

4. Over a medium-high heat, add the olive oil to a frying pan or wok and heat for 2–3 minutes. Add the tofu and fry for 3 minutes on each side until golden. Remove the tofu from the pan on to a plate or kitchen paper.

5. Reduce the heat to medium and add the spring onions and garlic. Cook for 1 minute, stirring the whole time. Add 200ml of water and the soy sauce and bring to a simmer.

6. Place 1 tbsp of cornflour and 2 tbsp of water into a bowl and stir.

7. Put the tofu back in the pan or wok and cook for a further 8 minutes. Add the cornflour mixture and stir until it is thickened.

8. Remove from the heat and drizzle with the peanut or sesame oil. Serve with wholewheat noodles, if desired.

Chicken and Chickpea Curry

This one-pot recipe is very straightforward and packed with protein, vitamins, minerals, fibre and antioxidants. I use chicken thighs in this curry as they are an excellent source of protein, crucial for muscle growth, repair and overall body function. They provide essential vitamins and minerals like B vitamins, including niacin and B12, iron and zinc, which play vital roles in energy production, immune function and overall health.

Chickpeas are a rich source of nutrients, especially protein and dietary fibre. They also have potential benefits for the maintenance of gut health by improving intestinal integrity and serving as a source of energy for the gut bacteria. Moreover, chickpea consumption has been found to possess anticancer, anti-inflammatory and antioxidant activity.

I like to use more than one spice in a recipe where I can, and cardamom is one of my favourites. Cardamom is known as the 'queen of the spices' and belongs to the same spice family as ginger. It's cultivated in India, Sri Lanka and Central America and has been used in culinary and traditional medicine practices since ancient times. It has warming properties, like cinnamon, nutmeg, clove and ginger. Cumin is the second spice I use in the curry – it is rich in antioxidants, including flavonoids that help to neutralize harmful free radicals that can damage cells and contribute to chronic diseases. Cumin also contains compounds that may reduce inflammation, potentially easing symptoms of inflammatory conditions like arthritis.

SERVES 4

- 2 tbsp extra virgin olive oil
- 4 boneless, skinless chicken thighs
- 2 red onions, chopped
- 3cm fresh ginger root, grated
- 2 garlic cloves, finely chopped
- 50g ground almonds
- 1 tsp cumin
- 1 tsp cardamom
- 2 x 400g tins chickpeas, drained
- 400ml coconut milk
- 120ml water
- Freshly ground black pepper

1. Over a medium-high heat, heat 1 tbsp of the olive oil in a large casserole dish. Add the chicken and brown for 4 minutes on each side. Set aside on a separate plate.

2. Add the remaining 1 tbsp of olive oil to the casserole dish, add the onions and cook for 5 minutes until softened.

3. Add the ginger and garlic and cook for a further 3 minutes.

4. Add the almonds, cumin and cardamom, stir and cook for 1 minute.

5. Add the chickpeas, coconut milk and water, bring to a simmer, then place the chicken on top of the curry. Cover with a lid and simmer for 18 minutes, stirring occasionally.

6. Once cooked, remove the chicken and shred it, then add back to the curry and stir. Season with freshly ground black pepper and serve with whole-grain rice.

Chilli Pepper Cod

Cod is high in protein while being low in fat and calories. It is a good source of the B vitamins, especially vitamin B12, which plays an important role in forming red blood cells and DNA.

Chilli peppers can influence both the immune system and gut health, primarily through the actions of capsaicin and other bioactive compounds. Capsaicin can affect the gut microbiota and potentially boost our beneficial bacteria and short-chain fatty acid (SCFA) production while also modulating immune responses.

SCFAs produced by gut bacteria can help regulate the immune system, protect the intestinal barrier and aid communication between the gut and the brain. Capsaicin can influence the activity of immune cells, potentially promoting a more balanced immune response. It may also help to reduce gut inflammation by inhibiting the production of pro-inflammatory cytokines and decreasing the abundance of certain bacteria associated with inflammation.

Note – while chilli peppers can be beneficial to health, it is important to consume them in moderation as some people can experience digestive side effects, such as heartburn or indigestion, especially those with pre-existing digestive conditions.

SERVES 4

- 1 red onion, finely chopped
- 1 yellow pepper, deseeded and sliced
- 1 red pepper, deseeded and sliced
- 1 tsp fennel seeds, crushed
- 3 tbsp extra virgin olive oil
- 2 garlic cloves, sliced
- 400g tin chopped tomatoes
- 1 tsp smoked paprika
- 4 x 120g cod fillets
- 1 red chilli, chopped
- Freshly ground black pepper
- Sea salt

1. Preheat the oven to 190°C/170°C fan/gas mark 5.

2. In a roasting tray, add the onion, peppers and crushed fennel seeds, and drizzle with 2 tbsp of the olive oil.

3. Place in the oven and cook for 18–20 minutes until the vegetables are softened.

4. Add the garlic, tomatoes and smoked paprika and cook for a further 15 minutes.

5. Place the cod fillets on top of the vegetables, drizzle over the remaining 1 tbsp of olive oil and scatter the chilli on top. Cook for 8 minutes or until the cod is fully cooked.

6. Season with freshly ground black pepper and sea salt, if desired.

Potato, Spinach and Chickpea Stew

Spinach is a good source of both soluble and insoluble fibre, which is crucial for digestive health and helps to regulate bowel movements, prevent constipation and promote a healthy gut microbiome. This nutritious leafy green vegetable contains sugar called sulfoquinovose, which acts as a prebiotic, nourishing our beneficial gut bacteria and helping to create a balanced and diverse microbiome, which is essential for optimal digestion and overall health.

Gut-healthy new potatoes contain resistant starch, a type of prebiotic fibre that ferments in the large intestine, feeding beneficial gut bacteria. This fermentation produces SCFAs, such as butyrate, which are crucial for colon cell health and have anti-inflammatory effects. SCFAs, particularly butyrate, help reduce inflammation in the gut, potentially lowering the risk of conditions like irritable bowel syndrome. By supporting a healthy gut microbiome, new potatoes indirectly contribute to immune system regulation as the gut plays a crucial role in immune response.

Ginger root is a great addition to this plant-based stew as it offers potential benefits for both immune system support and gut health due to its anti-inflammatory and antioxidant properties. It can aid digestion, reduce inflammation in the gastrointestinal tract and potentially strengthen the immune system by reducing the risk of infections. Furthermore, ginger contains compounds like gingerol, which has anti-inflammatory effects and can help combat free radicals. It may also positively influence gut microbiota composition, potentially contributing to a healthier gut environment, which is associated with improved immune function.

SERVES 4

- 250g new potatoes, halved
- 1 tbsp extra virgin olive oil
- 1 red onion, finely chopped
- 2cm fresh ginger root, finely chopped
- 2 garlic cloves, finely chopped
- 1 tsp turmeric
- 1 tsp ground cumin
- 2 x 400g tins chopped tomatoes
- 150ml water
- 400g tin chickpeas
- 200g baby spinach leaves, chopped
- Freshly ground black pepper

1. Over a medium-high heat bring a large saucepan of water to the boil.

2. Add the new potatoes and cook for 8 minutes, drain and set aside.

3. Over a medium heat, add the olive oil to a large pan and add the onion. Cook for 5 minutes until softened.

4. Add the ginger, garlic, turmeric and cumin and cook for a further 2 minutes.

5. Add the tomatoes, new potatoes and water, and bring to a simmer. Cook for 25 minutes.

6. Add the chickpeas and baby spinach and cook for a further 3–5 minutes until the spinach is wilted.

7. Season with freshly ground black pepper.

Beet It Burgers

These delicious plant-based burgers are made with beetroot, which is rich in fibre and beneficial compounds that can positively impact both the immune system and gut health. Beetroot provides both soluble and insoluble fibre, while compounds like betalains may act as antioxidants supporting our heath. These positive benefits can contribute to overall immune function and optimal digestive health.

Black beans are beneficial for both our immune system and gut health due to their high fibre content and ability to promote a healthy gut microbiome. The fibre in black beans, particularly resistant starch, ferments in the colon and produces SCFAs that reduce inflammation and support gut health. This, in turn, can strengthen the immune system and potentially help prevent gut-associated diseases. Research has indicated that black bean consumption can change the gut microbiome by increasing the beneficial gut bacteria while decreasing the gut bacteria which is associated with inflammation. Black beans also provide essential nutrients like folate, iron and zinc, which are crucial for immune cell development and function.

I use hazelnuts in this recipe, and they are a good source of vitamins and minerals that play a crucial role in immune function, such as vitamin E, zinc and copper, which are important for a healthy immune response. Hazelnuts contain polyphenols, which can benefit gut health by fuelling our beneficial bacteria and potentially increasing their numbers, leading to the production of SCFAs that are beneficial for both gut and overall health. Furthermore, the antioxidants found in hazelnuts can help combat inflammation and potentially reduce the risk of infections and illnesses.

SERVES 4

- 1 red onion, sliced
- 3 medium-sized beetroots, cooked
- 1 tsp ground cumin
- 1 tsp smoked paprika
- 400g tin black beans, drained
- 50g hazelnuts, chopped
- 2 tbsp extra virgin olive oil

1. Add the onion, beetroots, cumin, paprika, beans and hazelnuts to a food processor and blitz until smooth. Be careful not to overdo the blitzing as you risk the mixture becoming too soft.

2. Add the olive oil to a pan and heat over a medium heat.

3. Carefully form the mixture into 4 patties and transfer them to the pan.

4. Cook for 4–5 minutes and then turn the patties.

5. Cook for a further 4–5 minutes until the burgers are firm and are hot in the middle.

Tofu Pumpkin Curry

Tofu is a popular food derived from soya, which is made by curdling fresh soya milk, pressing it into a solid block and then cooling it, in much the same way that traditional dairy cheese is made by curdling and solidifying milk. It is very versatile and can be cooked in many different ways to change its texture from smooth and soft to crisp and crunchy. Tofu is high in plant compounds and other nutrients that can help reduce inflammation in the body. Inflammation is a natural process, but chronic inflammation can weaken the immune system and increase your risk of numerous health concerns.

Pumpkins are a great source of antioxidant vitamins A, C and E as well as immune-nourishing zinc, selenium and magnesium. It is also rich in fibre and other health-promoting antioxidants, such as lutein and zeaxanthin. Pumpkin also contains tryptophan, an amino acid that can help improve sleep.

This recipe also contains broccoli, which is high in vitamin C and other antioxidants that support our immune system. These antioxidants and anti-inflammatory compounds may also help protect against cell damage that can lead to cancer. Broccoli contains glucosinolates, which the body can convert into cancer-fighting compounds like sulforaphane. In addition, research shows that kaempferol, a flavonoid in broccoli, demonstrates strong anti-inflammatory capacity and could potentially help reduce inflammation.

SERVES 4

- 1 tbsp olive oil
- 300g tofu, drained and cut into 2.5cm cubes
- 150g broccoli, cut into small pieces
- 250g pumpkin, cut into 2.5cm cubes
- 1 tsp cumin seeds
- 1 tsp coriander seeds
- 400ml coconut milk
- ½ tsp red curry paste
- 1 tbsp fish sauce
- 1 lemongrass stalk, finely chopped
- 150g spinach

1. Add the olive oil to a large pan or wok, and over a medium-high heat fry the tofu, turning frequently until golden brown. Remove from the pan and set aside.

2. Add the broccoli and pumpkin to the pan with the cumin seeds and coriander seeds. Cook for 1–2 minutes, then add the coconut milk, red curry paste, fish sauce and lemongrass. Stir well and leave to simmer for 15–20 minutes until the vegetables are softened.

3. Add the spinach and tofu, stirring well. Cook until the spinach is wilted.

4. Serve with whole-grain rice.

Sweet Treats

Lemon and Blueberry Pancakes

Wholemeal flour is rich in fibre and various bioactive compounds that can significantly benefit both the immune system and gut health. The fibre in the flour supports our gut microbiome, which in turn plays a crucial role in immune function. The fibre can help slow down digestion, maintain stable blood-sugar levels and help us feel fuller for longer.

Blueberries are delicious and are very beneficial for both our immune system and gut health due to their high antioxidant and fibre content. They act as prebiotics and 'feed' our beneficial gut bacteria, and they can help to reduce inflammation and improve immune and gut health.

Lemon zest, derived from the outer layer of the lemon peel, can positively impact both the immune system and gut health due to its rich content of nutrients and bioactive compounds. It contains vitamin C, fibre and D-limonene, which contributes to immune function and digestive health, and may help to reduce inflammation. Research suggests that lemon peel, which includes the zest, may possess antimicrobial and antifungal properties, potentially helping to inhibit the growth of harmful microorganisms.

SERVES 4

- 180g wholemeal flour
- 1 tsp baking powder
- ½ tsp bicarbonate of soda
- ½ tsp sea salt
- 4 eggs
- 300ml milk of choice
- 100g natural Greek yoghurt
- 2 tbsp mild olive oil
- ½ tsp vanilla extract
- Zest of 1 lemon
- 400g blueberries
- 2 tsp maple syrup (optional)

1. Add the flour, baking powder, bicarbonate of soda and sea salt to a large bowl and mix.

2. In a second large bowl, add the eggs, milk, yoghurt, 1 tbsp of the mild olive oil, vanilla extract and lemon zest, and mix until smooth.

3. Combine the flour mixture and egg mixture, and stir to mix.

4. Over a medium-low heat, add the remaining 1 tbsp of mild olive oil to a frying pan, and gently heat.

5. With a ladle, add a ladleful of batter to the pan. Cook for 2 minutes until golden, flip, then cook the other side for 1 minute. Once cooked, set aside on a plate.

6. Repeat the process until all the batter is used.

7. Top the pancakes with the blueberries and serve warm. Drizzle with maple syrup, if desired.

Peanut Butter and Hazelnut Cookies

Peanuts are nutrient-rich and provide numerous essential micronutrients, including magnesium, iron and zinc as well as copper. They are also a source of vitamins including the B group and vitamin E. Additionally, peanut butter is a rich source of fat, including oleic acid, a healthy monounsaturated fat that has been linked to several health benefits, including improved insulin sensitivity (how responsive your cells are to insulin). Peanut butter is also a good source of fibre, which helps support gut health and digestive transit as well as managing appetite by improving satiety levels.

Hazelnuts are a rich source of vitamins and minerals like vitamin E, manganese and copper. Additionally, they have a high content of omega-6 and omega-9 fatty acids and may help prevent and decrease inflammation due to their high concentrations of healthy fats. Hazelnuts are rich in phenolic compounds that have been shown to exert antioxidant properties, which can help to support our health.

MAKES 12 COOKIES

- 120g peanut butter, no added sugar
- 125ml maple syrup
- 3 tbsp coconut oil
- 90g hazelnuts, chopped
- 120g spelt flour
- ½ tsp bicarbonate of soda

1. Preheat the oven to 180°C/160°C fan/gas mark 4. Line a baking sheet with baking paper.

2. Add the peanut butter, maple syrup, coconut oil and hazelnuts to a bowl, and mix well.

3. In a separate bowl, add the flour and bicarbonate of soda, and mix. Then add to the peanut butter mixture, and mix well.

4. Shape the dough into 12 individual balls and arrange on the baking sheet, making sure there is enough space between each. Flatten the balls to about 5mm thick and place in the oven for 12 minutes or until golden.

These cookies can keep in an airtight container for 3–5 days.

Pecan and Date Balls

Pecans are delicious and can help support both gut and immune health due to their rich nutrient profile. They are a good source of fibre, which promotes healthy digestion and supports the growth of beneficial gut bacteria. The fibre also helps regulate bowel movements and prevent constipation. Additionally, pecans contain various vitamins and minerals, such as magnesium, calcium, vitamin E and zinc, which have anti-inflammatory properties. These properties can help modulate the immune response and reduce inflammation in the body.

Dates are a good source of both soluble and insoluble fibre, containing prebiotic fibre, which acts as fuel for our beneficial gut bacteria, supporting a balanced gut microbiome. This can lead to improved digestion, better nutrient absorption and enhanced overall gut health. Research also suggests that dates may help to reduce the risk of certain colon-related issues due to their high fibre and polyphenol content.

SWEET TREATS

MAKES 10 BALLS

- 100g pecans
- 50g cashews, unsalted
- 200g dates, pitted
- 50g desiccated coconut

1. Add the pecans and cashews to a food processor and blitz until the nuts are a little crushed.

2. Add the dates and blitz until the mixture is like a dough.

3. Shape the dough into 10 balls and roll them in the desiccated coconut, coating them all over.

4. Pop into the fridge for 2 hours.

Warm Cinnamon Apple Pudding

Apples offer significant benefits for both gut health and the immune system due to their fibre and polyphenol content. Pectin, a type of fibre in apples, acts as a prebiotic, nourishing beneficial gut bacteria and promoting a healthy gut microbiome. This improved gut health can promote our ability to absorb nutrients, decrease inflammation and potentially strengthen immunity. In addition, apples contain antioxidants and vitamin C, which can further support immune health and protect against cell damage that could lead to illness and disease.

The fibre in raisins acts as a prebiotic and nourishes our beneficial gut bacteria, which can lead to a more balanced and diverse gut microbiome that is crucial for overall digestive health, immunity and well-being. Some compounds in raisins, such as phenolic acids, have anti-inflammatory effects and may help to reduce inflammation in the gut and promote a healthier intestinal environment.

Cinnamon inhibits the growth of harmful bacteria like **Salmonella** *and* **Listeria** *as well as the yeast* **Candida***, which can cause digestive issues and potentially contribute to autoimmune diseases. This tasty spice can also help to restore balance to the gut microbiome by acting as a prebiotic, and its anti-inflammatory compounds may help reduce inflammation in the gut.*

SWEET TREATS

SERVES 4

- 2 tbsp coconut oil, melted
- 4 large red apples, cored and cut into wedges
- 80g raisins
- 2 tsp ground cinnamon
- 2 tbsp chopped almonds

1. Preheat the oven to 160°C/140°C fan/gas mark 3.

2. With a small amount of coconut oil, brush the base of a dish or tin.

3. Place the apple slices into the dish or tin and pour over the remaining coconut oil.

4. Sprinkle over the raisins and cinnamon and place in the oven for 15 minutes.

5. Remove from the oven and scatter over the chopped almonds.

6. Turn the oven up to 180°C/160°C fan/gas mark 4 and cook for 10 minutes or until starting to brown.

7. Serve with yoghurt of choice – I like coconut yoghurt or natural Greek yoghurt with this pudding.

Fruit and Nut Chocolate

Coconut oil contains medium-chain triglycerides, which may support the growth of beneficial gut bacteria. Some research suggests coconut oil may help strengthen the gut barrier, potentially reducing leaky gut and preventing harmful substances from entering the bloodstream. Coconut oil is also a good source of lauric acid, which is converted into monolaurin and has potent antiviral, antibacterial and antifungal properties.

Raw cacao is packed with micronutrients, antioxidants and prebiotic fibre, which promote gut health and immune function. Its powerful antioxidants, like flavonols (a type of flavonoid), can provide several health benefits, such as helping to reduce inflammation in the gut and support a healthier environment for digestion. Cacao is also a source of minerals like iron and zinc, which are essential for a healthy immune system. It can even improve our mood due to several compounds it contains, including tryptophan, phenylethylamine and serotonin precursors. These compounds can encourage the release of 'feel-good' hormones like serotonin, endorphins and dopamine, which are associated with happiness and well-being. It is also a good source of magnesium, which can help calm the nervous system, reduce stress and anxiety, and promote good mood.

MAKES APPROXIMATELY 20 PIECES

- 100g coconut oil
- 100g butter
- 2 tbsp raw cacao or unsweetened cocoa powder
- 4 tsp maple syrup
- 50g sultanas or raisins
- 50g chopped nuts

1. Line a baking sheet with baking paper.

2. Over a low heat, melt the coconut oil and butter in a pan.

3. Add the raw cacao or cocoa powder and maple syrup, and stir well.

4. Pour the chocolate mixture on to the baking paper and scatter over the sultanas or raisins and chopped nuts.

5. Place in the freezer for 30 minutes until it is firm to the touch.

6. Remove from the freezer and cut into pieces.

This will keep up to 3 days in an airtight container in the fridge.

Acknowledgements

The Immunity Plan is the result of several people's hard work, support and reassurance and could simply not have been written without this.

Firstly, to Corinna Bolino, senior commissioning editor at Penguin Michael Joseph, for giving me this incredible opportunity and providing me with the invaluable guidance and support to write this book. I am so grateful and fortunate to be able to work with you. To my copy-editor DeAndra Lupu and editorial manager Katya Browne, for your continual patience during the editing process, and to the whole Pathways team for all your guidance, ideas and support, which has allowed me to bring this book to readers – thank you.

Hannah Weatherill, my agent at Watson Little, this book would not have been written without your tenacity, hard work and guidance – right through from the book proposal stage to publication. Working with you is a joy.

To Luke Speed at Insight Management, who I have known for 30 years since we were students at Warwick Uni – my writing career would not have happened without your support and guidance, thank you.

A big thank you to my family and close friends (you know who you are!) for their endless reassurance and positivity while I burrowed myself away writing for many months. I am so grateful for having you all in my life.

Finally, to my children, Beatrix and Albert – you are both incredibly special and bring me so much joy and happiness and have provided me with the greatest sense of purpose.

References

INTRODUCTION

1. Derek M. Griffith, Garima Sharma, Christopher S. Holliday, Okechuku K. Enyia, Matthew Valliere, Andrea R. Semlow, Elizabeth C. Stewart and Roger Scott Blumenthal, 'Men and COVID-19: A biopsychosocial approach to understanding sex differences in mortality and recommendations for practice and police interventions', cdc.gov (16 July 2020).
2. Maunil K. Desai and Roberta Diaz Brinton, 'Autoimmune disease in women: Endocrine transition and risk across the lifespan', *Frontiers in Endocrinology (Lausanne)*, 10:265 (2019).

1. IMMUNE SYSTEM BASICS

1. Ingrid Fricke-Galindo and Ramcés Falfán-Valencia, 'Genetics insight for COVID-19 susceptibility and severity: A review', *Frontiers in Immunology*, 12 (2021), 622176.
2. Lindsay B. Nicholson, 'The immune system', *Essays in Biochemistry*, 60:3 (2016), 275–301.
3. Isabelle Wolowczuk, Claudie Verwaerde, Odile Viltart, Anne Delanoye, Myriam Delacre, Bruno Pot and Corinne Grangette, 'Feeding our immune system: Impact on metabolism', *Clinical & Developmental Immunology*, (2008), 639803.
4. Diane Mathis and Steven E. Shoelson, 'Immunometabolism: an Emerging Frontier', *Nature Reviews Immunology*, 11 (2011), 81–83.

2. THE AUTOIMMUNITY CRISIS

1. 'Autoimmune diseases', niaid.nih.gov (20 March 2025).

REFERENCES

2. Nathalie Conrad, Shivani Misra, Jan Y. Verbakel, Geert Verbeke, Geert Molenberghs, Peter N. Taylor, Justin Mason, Naveed Sattar, John J. V. McMurray, Iain B. McInnes, Kamlesh Khunti and Geraldine Cambridge, 'Incidence, prevalence, and co-occurrence of autoimmune disorders over time and by age, sex, and socioeconomic status: A population-based cohort study of 22 million individuals in the UK', *Lancet*, 401:10391 (2023), 1878–1890.
3. Syreen Goulmamine, Sarah Chew and Irene O. Aninye, 'Autoimmune health crisis: An inclusive approach to addressing disparities in women in the United States', *International Journal of Environmental Research and Public Health*, 21:10 (2024), 1339.
4. Carlo Perricone and Yehuda Shoenfeld (eds), *Mosaic of Autoimmunity: The Novel Factors of Autoimmune Diseases* (Academic Press, 2019).
5. Juan-Manuel Anaya, Adriana Rojas-Villarraga and Yehuda Shoenfeld, 'From the Mosaic of Autoimmunity to the Autoimmune Tautology', in *Autoimmunity: From Bench to Bedside [Internet]*, eds Juan-Manuel Anaya, Yehuda Schoenfeld, Adriana Rojas-Villarraga, et al. (El Rosario University Press, 2013).
6. Aristo Vojdani, Michael K. Pollard and Andrew W. Campbell, 'Environmental triggers and autoimmunity', *Autoimmune Diseases*, (2014).
7. 'Rheumatoid arthritis: How common is it?', cks.nice.org.uk (April 2025).
8. 'Lupus', nhsinform.scot (22 February 2023).
9. 'Lupus', nhs.uk (19 July 2023).
10. Francesca Ragusa, Poupak Fallahi, Giusy Elia, Debora Gonnella, Sabrina Rosaria Paparo, Claudia Giusti, Leonid P. Churilov, Silvia Martina Ferrari and Alessandro Antonelli, 'Hashimoto's thyroiditis: Epidemiology, pathogenesis, clinic, and therapy', *Best Practice & Research Clinical Endocrinology & Metabolism*, 33:6 (2019).
11. Jasleen Kaur and Ishwarlal Jialal, *Hashimoto Thyroiditis* (StatPearls Publishing, 2020).
12. Mike Watts, 'Type 1 diabetes', diabetes.co.uk (29 October 2023).
13. 'Sjögren's syndrome', nhsinform.scot (21 February 2025).
14. Roberta Mazzone, Clemens Zwergel, Marco Artico, Samanta Taurone, Massimo Ralli, Antonio Greco and Antonello Mai, 'The emerging role of epigenetics in human autoimmune disorders', *Clinical Epigenetics*, 11:1 (2019), 1–15.

15. J. E. Blalock, 'The immune system as a sensory organ', *Journal of Immunology*, 132:3 (1984), 1067–1070.
16. DeLisa Fairweather and Noel R. Rose, 'Women and autoimmune diseases', nc.cdc.gov (November 2004).
17. Mimi Ghosh, Marta Rodriguez-Garcia and Charles R. Wira, 'The immune system in menopause: Pros and cons of hormone therapy', *Journal of Steroid Biochemistry and Molecular Biology*, 142 (2014), 171–175.
18. Maunil K. Desai and Roberta Diaz Brinton, 'Autoimmune disease in women: Endocrine transition and risk across the lifespan'.
19. Kassem Sharif, Abdulla Watad, Louis Coplan, Benjamin Lichtbroun, Alec Krosser, Michael Lichtbroun, Nicola Luigi Bragazzi, Howard Amital, Arnon Afek and Yehuda Schoenfeld, 'The role of stress in the mosaic of autoimmunity: An overlooked association', *Autoimmunity Reviews*, 17:10 (2018), 967–983.
20. Elena Philippou and Elena Nikiphorou, 'Are we really what we eat? Nutrition and its role in the onset of rheumatoid arthritis', *Autoimmunity Reviews*, 17:11 (2018), 1074–1077.
21. Mathilde Versini, Pierre-Yves Jeandel, Eric Rosenthal and Yehuda Shoenfeld, 'Obesity in autoimmune diseases: not a passive bystander', *Autoimmunity Reviews*, 13:9 (2014), 981–1000.
22. Selma P. Wiertsema, Jeroen van van Bergenhenegouwen, Johan Garssen and Leon M. J. Knippels, 'The interplay between the gut microbiome and the immune system in the context of infectious diseases throughout life and the role of nutrition in optimizing treatment strategies', *Nutrients*, 13:3 (2021), 886.
23. Alessio Fasano, 'Leaky gut and autoimmune diseases', *Clinical Reviews in Allergy & Immunology*, 42:1 (2012), 71–78.
24. Oded Shamriz and Yehuda Shoenfeld, 'Infections: a double-edge sword in autoimmunity', *Current Opinion in Rheumatology*, 30:4 (2018), 365–372.
25. Michael Ehrenfeld, Angela Tincani, Laura Andreoli, Marco Cattalini, Assaf Greenbaum, Darja Kanduc, Jaume Alijotas-Reig, Vsevolod Zinserling, Natalia Semenova, Howard Amital and Yehuda Shoenfeld, 'Covid-19 and autoimmunity', *Autoimmunity Reviews*, 19:8 (2020), 102597.

REFERENCES

26. 'Infectious mononucleosis', bestpractice.bmj.com (16 November 2021).
27. 'Infectious mononucleosis (glandular fever)', cks.nice.org.uk (November 2024).

3. ALLERGIES AND INFECTIONS

1. S. A. Alduraywish, C. J. Lodge, B. Campbell, K. J. Allen, B. Erbas, A. J. Lowe and S. C. Dharmage, 'The march from early life food sensitization to allergic disease: A systematic review and meta-analyses of birth cohort studies', *Allergy*, 71:1 (2016), 77–89.
2. Selene K. Bantz, Zhou Zhu and Tao Zheng, 'The atopic march: Progression from atopic dermatitis to allergic rhinitis and asthma', *Journal of Clinical & Cellular Immunology*, 5:2 (2014), 202.
3. Sinéad Máire Langan, Amy R. Mulick, Charlotte E. Rutter, Richard J. Silverwood, Innes Asher, Luis García-Marcos, Eamon Ellwood, Karen Bissell, Chen-Yuan Chiang, Asma El Sony, Philippa Ellwood, Guy B. Marks, Kevin Mortimer, A. Elena Martínez-Torres, Eva Morales, Virginia Perez-Fernandez, Steven Robertson, Hywel C. Williams, David P. Strachan and Neil Pearce, 'Trends in eczema prevalence in children and adolescents: A Global Asthma Network Phase I study', *Clinical & Experimental Allergy*, 53:3 (2023), 337–352.
4. 'Atopic dermatitis (eczema) triggers, allergens and irritants', allergyuk.org.
5. 'Atopic eczema', nhs.uk (6 September 2024).
6. Giuseppe di Mauro, Roberto Bernardini, Salvatore Barberi, Annalisa Capuano, Antonio Correra, Gian Luigi de' Angelis, Iride Dello Iacono, Maurizio de Martino, Daniele Ghiglioni, Dora Di Mauro, Marcello Giovannini, Massimo Landi, Gian Luigi Marseglia, Alberto Martelli, Vito Leonardo Miniello, Diego Peroni, Lucilla Ricottini Maria Giuseppa Sullo, Luigi Terracciano, Cristina Vascone, Elvira Verduci, Maria Carmen Verga and Elena Chiappini, 'Prevention of food and airway allergy: Consensus of the Italian Society of Preventive and Social Paediatrics, the Italian Society of Paediatric Allergy and Immunology, and Italian Society of Pediatrics', *World Allergy Organization Journal*, 9:1 (2016), 28.
7. Siti Muhamad Nur Husna, Hern-Tze Tina Tan, Norasnieda Md Shukri, Noor Suryani Mohd Ashari and Kah Keng Wong, 'Allergic rhinitis: A clinical and pathophysiological overview', *Frontiers in Medicine*, 7:9 (2022).

REFERENCES

8. G. K. Scadding, H. H. Kariyawasam, G. Scadding, R. Mirakian, R. J. Buckley, T. Dixon, S. R. Durham, S. Farooque, N. Jones, S. Leech, S. M. Nasser, R. Powell, G. Roberts, G. Rotiroti, A. Simpson, H. Smith and A. T. Clark, 'BSACI guideline for the diagnosis and management of allergic and non-allergic rhinitis' (Revised edition 2017; first edition 2007), *Clin Exp Allergy*, 47:7 (2017), 856–889.
9. Michael R. Perkin, Tara Bader, Alicja R. Rudnicka, David P. Strachan and Christopher G. Owen, 'Inter-relationship between rhinitis and conjunctivitis in allergic rhinoconjunctivitis and associated risk factors in rural UK children', *PLoS One*, 10:11 (2015).
10. Cezmi A. Akdis, Peter W. Hellings and Ioana Agache, *Global Atlas of Allergic Rhinitis and Chronic Rhinosinusitis* (European Academy of Allergy and Clinical Immunology, 2015).
11. Jonathan A. Bernstein, Joshua S. Bernstein, Richika Makol and Stephanie Ward, 'Allergic rhinitis: A review', *Journal of the American Medical Association*, 331:10 (2024), 866–877.
12. Syuji Yonekura, Yoshitaka Okamoto, Shigetoshi Horiguchi, Daiju Sakurai, Hideaki Chazono, Toyoyuki Hanazawa, Toru Okawa, Susumu Aoki and Akiyoshi Konno, 'Effects of aging on the natural history of seasonal allergic rhinitis in middle-aged subjects in South Chiba, Japan', *International Archives of Allergy & Immunology*, 157:1 (2012), 73–80.
13. Eileen M. Duggan, Jennifer Sturley, Anthony P. Fitzgerald, Ivan J. Perry and Jonathan O'B. Hourihane, 'The 2002–2007 trends of prevalence of asthma, allergic rhinitis and eczema in Irish schoolchildren', *Pediatric Allergy & Immunology*, 23:5 (2012), 464–471.
14. Shweta Akhouri and Steven A. House, *Allergic Rhinitis* (StatPearls Publishing, 2021).
15. Jurgita Saulyte, Carlos Regueira, Agustín Montes-Martínez, Polyna Khudyakov and Bahi Takkouche, 'Active or passive exposure to tobacco smoking and allergic rhinitis, allergic dermatitis, and food allergy in adults and children: a systematic review and meta-analysis', *PLoS Med*, 11:3 (2014).
16. G. K. Scadding, H. H. Kariyawasam, G. Scadding, R. Mirakian, R. J. Buckley, T. Dixon, S. R. Durham, S. Farooque, N. Jones, S. Leech, S. M. Nasser, R. Powell, G. Roberts, G. Rotiroti, A. Simpson, H. Smith and A. T. Clark, 'BSACI guideline for the diagnosis and management of allergic and non-allergic rhinitis'.

REFERENCES

17. Imène Gouia, Florence Joulain, Yi Zhang, Christopher L. Morgan and Asif H. Khan, 'Epidemiology of childhood asthma in the UK', *Journal of Asthma and Allergy*, 17 (2024), 1197–1205.
18. Jessica Reyes-Angel, Parisa Kaviany, Deepa Rastogi and Erick Forno, 'Obesity-related asthma in children and adolescents', *Lancet Child & Adolescent Health*, 6:10 (2022), 713–724.
19. Anne L. Wright, Debra A. Stern, Francine Kauffmann and Fernando D. Martinez, 'Factors influencing gender differences in the diagnosis and treatment of asthma in childhood: The Tucson Children's Respiratory Study', *Pediatric Pulmonology*, 41:4 (2006), 318–325.
20. M. R. Becklake and F. Kauffmann, 'Gender differences in airway behaviour over the human life span', *Thorax*, 54:12 (1999), 1119–1138.
21. Åsa Neuman, Cynthia Hohmann, Nicola Orsini, Göran Pershagen, Esben Eller, Henrik Fomsgaard Kjaer, Ulrike Gehring, Raquel Granell, John Henderson, Joachim Heinrich, Susanne Lau, Mark Nieuwenhuijsen, Jordi Sunyer, Christina Tischer, Maties Torrent, Ulrich Wahn, Alet H. Wijga, Magnus Wickman, Thomas Keil and Anna Bergström, 'Maternal smoking in pregnancy and asthma in preschool children: A pooled analysis of eight birth cohorts', *American Journal of Respiratory and Critical Care Medicine*, 186:10 (2012), 1037–1043.
22. Annabelle Bédard, Kate Northstone, A. John Henderson and Seif O. Shaheen, 'Maternal intake of sugar during pregnancy and childhood respiratory and atopic outcomes', *European Respiratory Journal*, 50:1 (2017).
23. Graham Devereux, Stephen W. Turner, Leone C. A. Craig, Geraldine McNeill, Sheelagh Martindale, Peter J. Harbour, Peter J. Helms and Anthony Seaton, 'Low maternal vitamin E intake during pregnancy is associated with asthma in 5-year-old children', *Am J Respir Crit Care Med*, 174:5 (2006), 499–507; Augusto A. Litonjua, Sheryl L. Rifas-Shiman, Ngoc P. Ly, Kelan G. Tantisira, Janet W. Rich-Edwards, Carlos A. Camargo Jr., Scott T. Weiss, Matthew W. Gillman and Diane R. Gold, 'Maternal antioxidant intake in pregnancy and wheezing illnesses in children at 2 y of age', *American Journal of Clinical Nutrition*, 84:4 (2006), 903–911; Hans Bisgaard, Jakob Stokholm, Bo L. Chawes, Nadja H. Vissing, Elin Bjarndóttir, Ann-Marie M. Schoos, Helene M. Wolsk, Tine M. Pedersen, Rebecca K. Vinding, Sunna Thorsteinsdóttir, Nilofar

V. Følsgaard, Nadia R. Fink, Jonathan Thorsen, Anders G. Pedersen, Johannes Waage, Morten A. Rasmussen, Ken D. Stark, Sjurdur F. Olsen and Klaus Bønnelykke, 'Fish oil-derived fatty acids in pregnancy and wheeze and asthma in offspring', *New England Journal of Medicine*, 375:26 (2016), 2530–2539.

24. Mette C. Tollånes, Dag Moster, Anne K. Daltveit and Lorentz M. Irgens, 'Cesarean section and risk of severe childhood asthma: A population-based cohort study', *Journal of Pediatrics*, 153:1 (2008), 112–116; Min-Sho Ku, Hai-Lun Sun, Ji-Nan Sheu, Hong-Shen Lee, Shun-Fa Yang and Ko-Huang Lue, 'Neonatal jaundice is a risk factor for childhood asthma: A retrospective cohort study', *Pediatr Allergy Immunol*, 23:7 (2012), 623–628; Jakob Stokholm, Astrid Sevelsted, Ulrik D. Anderson and Hans Bisgaard, 'Preeclampsia associates with asthma, allergy, and eczema in childhood', *Am J Respir Crit Care Med*, 195:5 (2017), 614–621.

25. Christine Cole Johnson, Edward L. Peterson, Christine L. M. Joseph, Dennis R. Ownby and Naomi Breslau, 'Birth weight and asthma incidence by asthma phenotype pattern in a racially diverse cohort followed through adolescence', *Journal of Asthma*, 52:10 (2015), 1006–1012.

26. Dara G. Torgerson, Elizabeth J. Ampleford, Grace Y. Chiu and W. James Gauderman, et al., 'Meta-analysis of genome-wide association studies of asthma in ethnically diverse North American populations', *Nature Genetics*, 43:9 (2011), 887–892.

27. 'Asthma', who.int (6 May 2024).

28. Scott H. Sicherer and Hugh A. Sampson, 'Food allergy: A review and update on epidemiology, pathogenesis, diagnosis, prevention, and management', *Journal of Allergy & Clinical Immunology*, 141:1 (2018), 41–58; Amy M. Branum and Susan L. Lukacs, 'Food allergy among children in the United States', *Pediatrics*, 124:6 (2009), 1549–1555; Ruchi S. Gupta, Elizabeth E. Springston, Manoj R. Warrier, Bridget Smith, Rajesh Kumar, Jacqueline Pongracic and Jane L. Holl, 'The prevalence, severity, and distribution of childhood food allergy in the United States', *Pediatrics*, 128:1 (2011), e9–e17.

29. J. J. Koplin, R. L. Peters, A-L Ponsonby, L. C. Gurrin, D. Hill, M. L. K. Tang, S. C. Dharmage and K. J. Allen, 'Increased risk of peanut allergy in infants of Asian-born parents compared to those of Australian-born parents', *Allergy*, 69:12 (2014), 1639–1647.

REFERENCES

30. Scott H. Sicherer and Hugh A. Sampson, 'Food allergy: A review and update on epidemiology, pathogenesis, diagnosis, prevention, and management', *J Allergy Clin Immunol*, 141:1 (2018), 41–58.
31. Mark Messina and Carina Venter, 'Recent surveys on food allergy prevalence', *Nutrition Today*, 55:1 (2020), 22–29.
32. Karen Stein, 'Severely restricted diets in the absence of medical necessity: The unintended consequences', *Journal of the Academy of Nutrition and Dietetics*, 114:7 (2014), 986–994.
33. Stefanie Sausenthaler, Sibylle Koletzko, Beate Schaaf, Irina Lehmann, Michael Borte, Olf Herbarth, Andrea von Berg, H-Erich Wichmann and Joachim Heinrich, 'Maternal diet during pregnancy in relation to eczema and allergic sensitization in the offspring at 2 years of age', *Am J Clin Nutr*, 85:2 (2008), 530–537; Karien Viljoen, Ricardo Segurado, John O'Brien, Celine Murrin, John Mehegan and Cecily C. Kelleher, 'Pregnancy diet and offspring asthma risk over a 10-year period: The Lifeways Cross Generation Cohort Study, Ireland', *BMJ Open*, 8:2 (2018), e017013; Christina E. West, Janet Dunstan, Suzi McCarthy, Jessica Metcalfe, Nina D'Vaz, Suzanne Meldrum, Wendy H. Oddy, Meri K. Tulic and Susan L. Prescott, 'Associations between maternal antioxidant intakes in pregnancy and infant allergic outcomes', *Nutrients*, 4:11 (2012), 1747–1758; J. A. Dunstan, C. West, S. McCarthy, J. Metcalfe, S. Meldrum, W. H. Oddy, M. K. Tulic, N. D'Vaz and S. L. Prescott, 'The relationship between maternal folate status in pregnancy, cord blood folate levels, and allergic outcomes in early childhood', *Allergy*, 67:1 (2012), 50–57; I. Romieu, M. Torrent, R. Garcia-Esteban, C. Ferrer, N Ribas-Fitó, J. M. Antó, and J. Sunyer, 'Maternal fish intake during pregnancy and atopy and asthma in infancy', *Clin Exp Allergy*, 37:4 (2007), 518–525; Y. Miyake, S. Sasaki, K. Tanaka and Y. Hirota, 'Consumption of vegetables, fruit, and antioxidants during pregnancy and wheeze and eczema in infants', *Allergy*, 65:6 (2010), 758–765; L. Chatzi, M. Torrent, I. Romieu, R. Garcia-Esteban, C. Ferrer, F. Vioque, M. Kogevinas and J. Sunyer, 'Mediterranean diet in pregnancy is protective for wheeze and atopy in childhood', *Thorax*, 63:6 (2008), 507–513; Alison N. Thorburn, Craig I. McKenzie, Sj Shen, Dragana Stanley, Laurence Macia, Linda J. Mason, Laura K. Roberts, Connie H. Y. Wong, Raymond Shim, Remy Robert, Nina Chevalier, Jian K. Tan, Eliana

Mariño, Rob J. Moore, Lee Wong, Malcolm J. McConville, Dedreia L. Tull, Lisa G. Wood, Vanessa E. Murphy, Joerg Mattes, Peter G. Gibson and Charles R. Mackay, 'Evidence that asthma is a developmental origin disease influenced by maternal diet and bacterial metabolites', *Nature Communications*, 6 (2015), 7320.

34. Rachelle A. Pretorius, Marie Bodinier, Susan L. Prescott and Debra J. Palmer, 'Maternal fiber dietary intakes during pregnancy and infant allergic disease', *Nutrients*, 11:8 (2019), 1767.

35. Alison N. Thorburn, Craig I. McKenzie, Sj Shen, Dragana Stanley, Laurence Macia, Linda J. Mason, Laura K. Roberts, Connie H. Y. Wong, Raymond Shim, Remy Robert, Nina Chevalier, Jian K. Tan, Eliana Mariño, Rob J. Moore, Lee Wong, Malcolm J. McConville, Dedreia L. Tull, Lisa G. Wood, Vanessa E. Murphy, Joerg Mattes, Peter G. Gibson and Charles R. Mackay, 'Evidence that asthma is a developmental origin disease influenced by maternal diet and bacterial metabolites', *Nat Commun*, 6 (2015), 7320.

36. Nour Baïz, Jocelyne Just, Julie Chastang, Anne Forhan, Blandine de Lauzon-Guillain, Anne-Marie Magnier and Isabella Annesi-Maesano, 'Maternal diet before and during pregnancy and risk of asthma and allergic rhinitis in children', *Allergy, Asthma and Clinical Immunology*, 15 (2019), 40.

37. Mark Messina and Carina Venter, 'Recent surveys on food allergy prevalence', *Nutrition Today*, 55:1 (2020), 22–29.

38. Angela J. Frodsham and Adrian V. S. Hill, 'Genetics of infectious diseases', *Human Molecular Genetics*, 13:2 (2004), R187–R194.

39. Devin J. Kenney, Aoife K. O'Connell, Jacquelyn Turcinovic, Paige Montanaro, Ryan M. Hekman, Tomokazu Tamura, Andrew R. Berneshawi, Thomas R. Cafiero, Salam Al Abdullatif, Benjamin Blum, Stanley I. Goldstein, Brigitte L. Heller, Hans P. Gertje, Esther Bullitt, Alexander J. Trachtenberg, Elizabeth Chavez, Evans Tuekam Nono, Catherine Morrison, Anna E. Tseng, Amira Sheikh, Susanna Kurnick, Kyle Grosz, Markus Bosmann, Maria Ericsson, Bertrand R. Huber, Mohsan Saeed, Alejandro B. Balazs, Kevin P. Francis, Alexander Klose, Neal Paragas, Joshua D. Campbell, John H. Connor, Andrew Emili, Nicholas A. Crossland, Alexander Ploss and Florian Douam, 'Humanized mice reveal a macrophage-enriched gene signature defining human lung tissue protection during SARS-CoV-2 infection', *Cell Reports*, 39:3 (2022), 110714.

REFERENCES

40. Philip C. Calder, Anitra C. Carr, Adrian F. Gombart and Manfred Eggersdorfer, 'Optimal nutritional status for a well-functioning immune system is an important factor to protect against viral infections', *Nutrients*, 12:4 (2020), 1181.

4. IMMUNOMETABOLISM

1. Sharon S. Evans, Elizabeth A. Repasky and Daniel T. Fisher, 'Fever and the thermal regulation of immunity: The immune system feels the heat', *Nature Reviews Immunology*, 15:6 (2015), 335–349.
2. Alexander Lercher, Hatoon Baazim and Andreas Bergthaler, 'Systemic immunometabolism: Challenges and opportunities', *Immunity*, 53:3 (2020), 496–509.
3. Joana Araújo, Jianwen Cai and June Stevens, 'Prevalence of optimal metabolic health in American adults: National Health and Nutrition Examination Survey 2009–2016', *Metabolic Syndrome & Related Disorders*, 17:1 (2019), 46–52.
4. Loretta DiPietro, Andrei Gribok, Michelle S. Stevens, Larry F. Hamm and William Rumpler, 'Three 15-min bouts of moderate postmeal walking significantly improves 24-h glycemic control in older people at risk for impaired glucose tolerance', *Diabetes Care*, 36:10 (2013), 3262–3268.
5. Jotham Suez, Tal Korem, David Zeevi, Gili Zilberman-Schapira, Christoph A. Thaiss, Ori Maza, David Israeli, Niv Zmora, Shlomit Gilad, Adina Weinberger, Yael Kuperman, Alon Harmelin, Ilana Kolodkin-Gal, Hagit Shapiro, Zamir Halpern, Eran Segal and Eran Elinav, 'Artificial sweeteners induce glucose intolerance by altering the gut microbiota', *Nature*, 514:7521 (2014), 181–186.
6. Daniela S. Valdes, Daniel So, Paul A. Gill and Nicole J. Kellow, 'Effect of dietary acetic acid supplementation on plasma glucose, lipid profiles, and body mass index in human adults: A systematic review and meta-analysis', *Journal of the Academy of Nutrition and Dietetics*, 121:5 (2021), 895–914.
7. G. A. Bray, K. K. Kim and J. P. H. Wilding, 'Obesity: A chronic relapsing progressive disease process. A position statement of the World Obesity Federation', *Obesity Reviews*, 18:7 (2017), 715–723.
8. Alessandro Federico, Elena D'Aiuto, Francesco Borriello, Giusi Barra, Antonietta Gerarda Gravina, Marco Romano and Raffaele De

Palma, 'Fat: A matter of disturbance for the immune system', *World Journal of Gastroenterology*, 16:38 (2010), 4762–4772.
9. Chrysi Koliaki, Maria Dalamaga and Stavros Liatis, 'Update on the obesity epidemic: After the sudden rise, is the upward trajectory beginning to flatten?', *Current Obesity Reports*, 12:4 (2023), 514–527.
10. Alessandro Federico, Elena D'Aiuto, Francesco Borriello, Giusi Barra, Antonietta Gerarda Gravina, Marco Romano and Raffaele De Palma, 'Fat: A matter of disturbance for the immune system'.
11. Karla E. Merz and Debbie C. Thurmond, 'Role of skeletal muscle in insulin resistance and glucose uptake', *Comprehensive Physiology*, 10:3 (2020), 785–809.

5. THE IMPORTANCE OF MICROBIOMES

1. Emily R. Leeming, Abigail J. Johnson, Tim D. Spector and Caroline I. Le Roy, 'Effect of diet on the gut microbiota: Rethinking intervention duration', *Nutrients*, 11:12 (2019), 2862.
2. Gregg E. Dinse, Christine G. Parks, Clarice R. Weinberg, Caroll A. Co, Jesse Wilkerson, Darryl C. Zeldin, Edward K. L. Chan and Frederick W. Miller, 'Increasing prevalence of antinuclear antibodies in the United States', *Arthritis & Rheumatology*, 72:6 (2020), 1026–1035; Mohammad G. Saklayen, 'The global epidemic of the metabolic syndrome', *Current Hypertension Reports*, 20:2 (2018), 12.
3. Yong Fan and Oluf Pedersen, 'Gut microbiota in human metabolic health and disease', *Nature Reviews Microbiology*, 19:1 (2021), 55–71; Thomas Hrncir, Lucia Hrncirova, Miloslav Kverka and Helena Tlaskalova-Hogenova, 'The role of gut microbiota in intestinal and liver diseases', *Lab Anim*, 53:3 (2019), 271–280.
4. Yun Kit Yeoh, Tao Zuo, Grace Chung-Yan Lui, Fen Zhang, Qin Liu, Amy Y. L. Li, Arthur C. K. Chung, Chun Pan Cheung, Eugene Y. K. Tso, Kitty S. C. Fung, Veronica Chan, Lowell Ling, Gavin Joynt, David Shu-Cheong Hui, Kai Ming Chow, Susanna So Shan Ng, Timothy Chun-Man Li, Rita W. Y. Ng, Terry C. F. Yip, Grace Lai-Hung Wong, Francis K. L. Chan, Chun Kwok Wong, Paul K. S. Chan and Siew C. Ng, 'Gut microbiota composition reflects disease severity and dysfunctional immune responses in patients with COVID-19', *Gut*, 70:4 (2021), 698–706.

REFERENCES

5. Aleksander D. Kostic, Dirk Gevers, Heli Silijander, Tommi Vatanen, Tuulia Hyötyläinen, Anu-Maaria Hämäläinen, Aleksandr Peet, Vallo Tillmann, Päivi Pöhö, Ismo Mattila, Harri Lähdesmäki, Eric A. Franzosa, Outi Vaarala, Marcus de Goffau, Hermie Harmsen, Jorma Llonen, Suvi M. Virtanen, Clary B. Clish, Matej Orešič, Curtis Huttenhower, Mikael Knip, DIABIMMUNE Study Group and Ramnik J. Xavier, 'The dynamics of the human infant gut microbiome in development and in progression toward type 1 diabetes', *Cell Host Microbe*, 17:2 (2015), 260–273.
6. Filip Scheperjans, Velma Aho, Pedro A. B. Pereira, Kaisa Koskinen, Lars Paulin, Eero Pekkonen, Elena Haapaniemi, Seppo Kaakkola, Johanna Eerola-Rautio, Marjatta Pohja, Esko Kinnunen, Kari Murros and Petri Auvinen, 'Gut microbiota are related to Parkinson's disease and clinical phenotype', *Movement Disorders*, 30:3 (2015), 350–358.
7. Yun Kit Yeoh, Tao Zuo, Grace Chung-Yan Lui, Fen Zhang, Qin Liu, Amy Y. L. Li, Arthur C. K. Chung, Chun Pan Cheung, Eugene Y. K. Tso, Kitty S. C. Fung, Veronica Chan, Lowell Ling, Gavin Joynt, David Shu-Cheong Hui, Kai Ming Chow, Susanna So Shan Ng, Timothy Chun-Man Li, Rita W. Y. Ng, Terry C. F. Yip, Grace Lai-Hung Wong, Francis K. L. Chan, Chun Kwok Wong, Paul K. S. Chan and Siew C. Ng, 'Gut microbiota composition reflects disease severity and dysfunctional immune responses in patients with COVID-19'.
8. Thomas Hrncir, 'Gut microbiota dysbiosis: Triggers, consequences, diagnostic and therapeutic options', *Microorganisms*, 10:3 (2022), 578.
9. Shunying Yu, Yibin Sun, Zinyu Shao, Yuqing Zhou, Yang Yu, Ziaoyi Kuai and Chunli Zhou, 'Leaky gut in IBD: Intestinal barrier–gut microbiota interaction', *Journal of Microbiology and Biotechnology*, 32:7 (2022), 825–834.
10. Mary Ellen Sanders, Daniel J. Merenstein, Gregor Reid, Glenn R. Gibson and Robert A. Rastall, 'Probiotics and prebiotics in intestinal health and disease: From biology to the clinic', *Nature Reviews Gastroenterology & Hepatology*, 16:10 (2019), 605–616.
11. Priya Nimish Deo and Revati Deshmukh, 'Oral microbiome: Unveiling the fundamentals', *Journal of Oral & Maxillofacial Pathology*, 23:1 (2019), 122–128.
12. Carlos M. Moreno, Ellie Boeree, Claudia M Tellez Freitas and K. Scott Weber, 'Immunomodulatory role of oral microbiota in inflammatory diseases and allergic conditions', *Front Allergy*, 4 (2023).

13. Lars Rydén, Kåre Buhlin, Eva Ekstrand, Ulf de Faire, Anders Gustafsson, Jacob Holmer, Barbro Kjellström, Bertil Lindahl, Anna Norhammar, Åke Nygren, Per Näsman, Nilminie Rathnayake, Elisabet Svenungsson and Björn Klinge, 'Periodontitis increases the risk of a first myocardial infarction: A report from the PAROKRANK Study', *Circulation*, 133:6 (2016), 576–583.
14. Maurizio S. Tonetti, Francesco D'Aiuto, Luigi Nibali, Ann Donald, Clare Storry, Mohamed Parkar, Jean Suvan, Aroon D. Hingorani, Patrick Vallance and John Deanfield, 'Treatment of periodontitis and endothelial function', *New England Journal of Medicine*, 356:9 (2007), 911–920.
15. Stephen S. Dominy, Casey Lynch, Florian Ermini, Malgorzata Benedyk, Agata Marczyk, Andrei Konradi, Mai Nguyen, Ursula Haditsch, Debasish Raha, Christina Griffin, Leslie J. Holsinger, Shirin Arastu-Kapur, Samer Kaba, Alexander Lee, Mark I. Ryder, Barbara Potempa, Piotr Mydel, Annelie Hellvard, Karina Adamowicz, Hatice Hasturk, Glenn D. Walker, Eric C. Reynolds, Richard L. M. Faull, Maurice A. Curtis, Mike Dragunow and Jan Potempa, 'Porphyromonas gingivalis in Alzheimer's disease brains: Evidence for disease causation and treatment with small-molecule inhibitors', *Science Advances*, 5:1 (2019).
16. Carlos M. Moreno, Ellie Boeree, Claudia M Tellez Freitas and K. Scott Weber, 'Immunomodulatory role of oral microbiota in inflammatory diseases and allergic conditions', *Front Allergy*, 4 (2023).
17. Kosuke Mima, Shuji Ogino, Shigeki Nakagawa, Hiroshi Sawayama, Koichi Kinoshita, Ryuichi Krashima, Takatsugu Ishimoto, Katsunori Imai, Masaaki Iwatsuki, Daisuke Hashimoto, Yoshifumi Baba, Yasuo Sakamoto, Yo-Ichi Yamashita, Naoya Yoshida, Akira Chikamoto, Takatoshi Ishikoand and Hideo Baba, 'The role of intestinal bacteria in the development and progression of gastrointestinal tract neoplasms', *Surgical Oncology*, 26:4 (2017), 368–376.

6. THE GOOD GUT HEALTH PLAN

1. Joshua Z. Goldenberg, Christina Yap, Lyubov Lytvyn, Carlvin Ka-Fung Lo, Jennifer Beardsley, Dominik Mertz and Bradley C. Johnston, 'Probiotics for the prevention of Clostridium difficile-associated diarrhea in adults and children', *Cochrane Database of Systematic Reviews*, 12:12 (2017).

REFERENCES

2. Glenn R. Gibson, Karen P. Scott, Robert A. Rastall, Kieran M. Tuohy, Arland Hotchkiss, Alix Dubert-Ferrandon, Melani Gareau, Eileen F. Murphy, Delphine Saulnier, Gunnar Loh, Sandra Macfarlane, Nathalie Delzenne, Yehuda Ringel, Gunhild Kozianowski, Robin Dickmann, Irene Lenoir-Wijnkoop, Carey Walker and Randal Buddington, 'Dietary prebiotics: Current status and new definition', *Food Science & Technology Bulletin: Functional Foods*, 7:1 (2010), 1–19.
3. Faraz Bishehsari, Emmeline Magno, Garth Swanson, Vishal Desai, Robin M. Voigt, Christopher B. Forsyth and Ali Keshavarzian, 'Alcohol and gut-derived inflammation', *Alcohol Research*, 38:2 (2017), 163–171.
4. Lucia Hrncirova, Tomas Hudcovic, Eliska Sukova, Vladimira Machova, Eva Trckova, Jan Krejsek and Tomas Hrncir, 'Human gut microbes are susceptible to antimicrobial food additives in vitro', *Folia Microbiologica (Praha)*, 64:4 (2019), 497–508.
5. Benoit Chassaing, Tom Van de Wiele, Jana De Bodt, Massimo Marzorati and Andrew T. Gewirtz, 'Dietary emulsifiers directly alter human microbiota composition and gene expression ex vivo potentiating intestinal inflammation', *Gut*, 66:8 (2017), 1414–1427.

7. HOW TO EAT FOR A BALANCED IMMUNE SYSTEM – MACRONUTRIENTS

1. Qiang Sun, Jia Li and Feng Gao, 'New insights into insulin: The anti-inflammatory effect and its clinical relevance', *World Journal of Diabetes*, 5:2 (2014), 89–96.
2. Christina L. Sherry, Stephanie S. Kim, Ryan N. Dilger, Laura L. Bauer, Morgan L. Moon, Richard I. Tapping, George C. Fahey Jr., Kelly A. Tappenden and Gregory G. Freund, 'Sickness behavior induced by endotoxin can be mitigated by the dietary soluble fiber, pectin, through up-regulation of IL-4 and Th2 polarization', *Brain, Behavior, and Immunity*, 24:4 (2010), 631–640.
3. Erica D. Sonnenburg, Samuel A. Smits, Mikhail Tikhonov, Steven K. Higginbottom, Ned S. Wingreen and Justin L. Sonnenburg, 'Diet-induced extinctions in the gut microbiota compound over generations', *Nature*, 529:7585 (2016), 212–215.
4. Umar Bacha, Muhammad Nasir, Sanaullah Iqbal and Aftab Ahmad Anjum, 'Nutraceutical, anti-inflammatory, and immune

modulatory effects of β-glucan isolated from yeast', *BioMed Research International*, (2017).

5. Joanne L. Slavin, 'Position of the American Dietetic Association: Health implications of dietary fiber', *Journal of the American Dietetic Association*, 108:10 (2008), 1716–1731; Stephanie Jew, Suhad S. AbuMweis and Peter J. H. Jones, 'Evolution of the human diet: Linking our ancestral diet to modern functional foods as a means of chronic disease prevention', *Journal of Medicinal Food*, 12:5 (2009), 925–934; Edward C. Deehan and Jens Walter, 'The fiber gap and the disappearing gut microbiome: Implications for human nutrition', *Trends in Endocrinology & Metabolism*, 27:5 (2016), 239–242.

6. Stephen J. D. O'Keefe, Jia V. Li, Leo Lahti, Junhai Ou, Franck Carbonero, Khaled Mohammed, Joram M. Posma, James Kinross, Elaine Wahl, Elizabeth Ruder, Kishore Vipperla, Vasudevan Naidoo, Lungile Mtshali, Sebastian Tims, Philippe G. B. Puylaert, James DeLany, Alyssa Krasinskas, Ann C. Benefiel, Hatem O. Kaseb, Keith Newton, Jeremy K. Nicholson, Willem M. de Vos, H. Rex Gaskins and Erwin G. Zoetendal, 'Fat, fibre and cancer risk in African Americans and rural Africans', *Nat Commun*, 6 (2015), 1–14.

7. Alison M. Stephen, Martine M-J Champ, Susan J. Cloran, Mathilde Fleith, Lilou van Lieshout, Heddie Mejborn and Victoria J. Burley, 'Dietary fibre in Europe: Current state of knowledge on definitions, sources, recommendations, intakes and relationships to health', *Nutrition Research Reviews*, 30:2 (2017), 149–190.

8. S. Boyd Eaton, 'The ancestral human diet: What was it and should it be a paradigm for contemporary nutrition?', *Proceedings of the Nutrition Society*, 65:1 (2006), 1–6.

9. Andrew Reynolds, Jim Mann, John Cummings, Nicola Winter, Evelyn Mete and Lisa Te Morenga, 'Carbohydrate quality and human health: A series of systematic reviews and meta-analyses', *Lancet*, 393:10170 (2019), 434–445.

10. Patrice D. Cani, Claude Knauf, Miguel A. Iglesias, Daniel J. Drucker, Nathalie M. Delzenne and Rémy Burcelin, 'Improvement of glucose tolerance and hepatic insulin sensitivity by oligofructose requires a functional glucagon-like peptide 1 receptor', *Diabetes*, 55:5 (2006), 1484–1490; P. D. Cani, S. Possemiers, T. Van de Wiele,

REFERENCES

Y. Guiot, A. Everard, O. Rottier, L. Geurts, D. Naslain, A. Neyrinck, D. M. Lambert, G. G. Muccioli and N. M. Delzenne, 'Changes in gut microbiota control inflammation in obese mice through a mechanism involving GLP-2-driven improvement of gut permeability', *Gut*, 58:8 (2009), 1091–1103; Audrey M. Neyrinck, Sam Possemiers, Céline Druart, Tom Van de Wiele, Fabienne De Backer, Patrice D. Cani, Yvan Larondelle and Nathalie M. Delzenne, 'Prebiotic effects of wheat arabinoxylan related to the increase in bifidobacteria, roseburia and bacteroides/prevotella in diet-induced obese mice', *PLoS One*, 6:6 (2011), e20944; Justin L. Sonnenburg and Fredrik Bäckhed, 'Diet–microbiota interactions as moderators of human metabolism', *Nature*, 535:7610 (2016), 56–64.

11. Mrinal Samtiya, Rotimi E. Aluko, Tejpal Dhewa and José Manuel Moreno-Rojas, 'Potential health benefits of plant food-derived bioactive components: An overview', *Foods*, 10:4 (2021), 839.
12. Sujuan Ding, Hongmei Jiang and Jun Fang, 'Regulation of immune function by polyphenols', *Journal of Immunology Research*, (2018).
13. Ibid.
14. Simona Bungau, Mohamed M. Abdel-Daim, Delia Mirela Tit, Esraa Ghanem, Shimpei Sato, Maiko Maruyama-Inoue, Shin Yamane and Kazuaki Kadonosono, 'Health benefits of polyphenols and carotenoids in age-related eye diseases', *Oxidative Medicine and Cellular Longevity*, (2019).
15. J. de Felippe Júnior, M. da Rocha e Silva Júnior, F. M. Maciel, A. de M. Soares and N. F. Mendes, 'Infection prevention in patients with severe multiple trauma with the immunomodulator beta 1-3 polyglucose (glucan)', *Surgery, Gynecology & Obstetrics*, 177:4 (1993), 383–388.
16. 'Can plant-based food swaps cut your risk of heart disease?', bhf.org.uk (15 January 2024).
17. Peng Li, Yu-Long Yin, Defa Li, Sung Wo Kim and Guoyao Wu, 'Amino acids and immune function', *British Journal of Nutrition*, 98:2 (2007), 237–252.
18. Jürgen Bauer, Gianni Biolo, Tommy Cederholm, Matteo Cesari, Alfonso J. Cruz-Jentoft, John E. Morley, Stuart Phillips, Cornel Sieber, Peter Stehle, Daniel Teta, Renuka Visvanathan, Elena Volpi and Yves

Boirie, 'Evidence-based recommendations for optimal dietary protein intake in older people: A position paper from the PROT-AGE Study Group', *Journal of the American Medical Directors Association*, 14:8 (2013), 542–559.
19. Maral Bishehkolaei and Yashwant Pathak, 'Influence of omega n-6/n-3 ratio on cardiovascular disease and nutritional interventions', *Human Nutrition & Metabolism*, 37 (2024), 200275.
20. Ibid.
21. G. C. Román, R. E. Jackson, R. Gadhia, A. N, Románand J. Reis, 'Mediterranean diet: The role of long-chain ω-3 fatty acids in fish; polyphenols in fruits, vegetables, cereals, coffee, tea, cacao and wine; probiotics and vitamins in prevention of stroke, age-related cognitive decline, and Alzheimer disease', *Revue Neurologique (Paris)*, 175:10 (2019), 724–741.
22. 'Fat: the facts', nhs.uk (14 April 2023).
23. Mike Watts, 'Trans fats', diabetes.co.uk (29 October 2023).

8. HOW TO EAT FOR A BALANCED IMMUNE SYSTEM – MICRONUTRIENTS

1. Jun-Man Hong, Jin-Hee Kim, Jae Seung Kang, Wang Jae Lee and Young-Il Hwang, 'Vitamin C is taken up by human T cells via sodium-dependent vitamin C transporter 2 (SVCT2) and exerts inhibitory effects on the activation of these cells in vitro', *Anatomy & Cell Biology*, 49:2 (2016), 88–98; Umar Shahbaz, Nazira Fatima, Samra Basharat, Asma Bibi, Ziaobin Yu, Muhammad Iftikhar Hussain and Maryam Nasrullah, 'Role of vitamin C in preventing of COVID-19 infection, progression and severity', *AIMS Microbiology*, 8:1 (2022), 108–124.
2. Ruben Manuel Luciano Colunga Biancatelli, Max Berrill, John D. Catravas and Paul E. Marik, 'Quercetin and vitamin C: An experimental, synergistic therapy for the prevention and treatment of SARS-CoV-2 related disease (COVID-19)', *Front Immunol*, 11 (2020), 1451.
3. Umar Shahbaz, Nazira Fatima, Samra Basharat, Asma Bibi, Ziaobin Yu, Muhammad Iftikhar Hussain and Maryam Nasrullah, 'Role of vitamin C in preventing of COVID-19 infection, progression and severity', *AIMS Microbiol*, 8:1 (2022), 108–124.

REFERENCES

4. Harri Hemilä and Elizabeth Chalker, 'Vitamin C for preventing and treating the common cold', *Cochrane Database of Systematic Reviews*, 1 (2013).
5. Umar Shahbaz, Nazira Fatima, Samra Basharat, Asma Bibi, Ziaobin Yu, Muhammad Iftikhar Hussain and Maryam Nasrullah, 'Role of vitamin C in preventing of COVID-19 infection, progression and severity', *AIMS Microbiol*, 8:1 (2022), 108–124.
6. Aneta Otocka-Kmiecik and Aleksandra Król, 'The role of vitamin C in two distinct physiological states: Physical activity and sleep', *Nutrients*, 12:12 (2020), 3908.
7. '5 A Day portion sizes', nhs.uk (19 July 2022).
8. 'B vitamins and folic acid', nhs.uk (3 August 2020).
9. Kathleen Mikkelsen, Lily Stojanovska, Monica Prakash and Vasso Apostolopoulos, 'The effects of vitamin B on the immune/cytokine network and their involvement in depression', *Maturitas*, 96 (2017), 58–71.
10. 'Causes: Vitamin B12 or folate deficiency anaemia', nhs.uk (20 February 2023).
11. 'Rickets and osteomalacia', 111.wales.nhs.uk (17 October 2025).
12. H. Verhagen, B. Buijsse B, E. Jansen and B. Bueno de Mesquita, 'The state of antioxidant affairs', *Nutrition Today*, 41:6 (2006), 244–250.
13. William S. Blaner, 'Vitamin A and Provitamin A Carotenoids', in *Present Knowledge in Nutrition*, eds Bernadette P. Marriott, Diane F. Birt, Virginia A. Stallings and Allison A. Yates (Wiley-Blackwell, 2020), pp. 73–91.
14. A. Catharine Ross, Benjamin H. Caballero, Robert J. Cousins, Katherine L. Tucker and Thomas R. Ziegler, *Modern Nutrition in Health and Disease* (Lippincott Williams & Wilkins, eleventh edition, 2012), pp. 260–277.
15. Zhiyi Huang, Yu Liu, Guangying Qi, David Brand and Song Guo Zheng, 'Role of vitamin A in the immune system', *Journal of Clinical Medicine*, 7:9 (2018), 258.
16. Sherry A. Tanumihardjo, Robert M. Russell, Charles B. Stephensen, Bryan M. Gannon, Neal E. Craft, Marjorie J. Haskell, Georg Lietz, Kerry Schulze and Daniel J. Raiten, 'Biomarkers of nutrition for development (BOND) – vitamin A review', *Journal of Nutrition*, 146:9 (2016), 1816S–1848S.
17. Min Xian Wang, Shwe Sin Win and Junxiong Pang, 'Zinc supplementation reduces common cold duration among healthy adults: A systematic review of randomized controlled trials with

micronutrients supplementation', *American Journal of Tropical Medicine & Hygiene*, 103:1 (2020), 86–99.
18. Muhammed Majeed, Kalyanam Nagabhushanam, Priji Prakasan and Lakshmi Mundkur, 'Can selenium reduce the susceptibility and severity of SARS-CoV-2?: A comprehensive review', *International Journal of Molecular Sciences*, 23:9 (2022), 4809.
19. Anna Velia Stazi and Biagino Trinti, 'Selenium status and over-expression of interleukin-15 in celiac disease and autoimmune thyroid diseases', *Annali dell'Istituto Superiore di Sanità*, 46:4 (2010), 389–399.
20. Sumel Ashique, Shubneesh Kumar, Afzal Hussain, Neeraj Mishra, Ashish Garg, B. H. Jaswanth Gowda, Arshad Farid, Gaurav Gupta, Kamal Dua and Farzad Taghizadeh-Hesary, 'A narrative review on the role of magnesium in immune regulation, inflammation, infectious diseases, and cancer', *Journal of Health, Population & Nutrition*, 42:1 (2023), 74.
21. Institute of Medicine, Food and Nutrition Board, *Dietary Reference Intakes: Calcium, Phosphorus, Magnesium, Vitamin D and Fluoride* (National Academy Press, 1997).
22. Dharam P. Chaudhary, Rajeshwar Sharma and Devi D. Bansal, 'Implications of magnesium deficiency in type 2 diabetes: A review', *Biological Trace Element Research*, 134:2 (2010), 119–129.
23. Robert K. Rude, 'Magnesium', in *Modern Nutrition in Health and Disease*, eds A. Catharine Ross, Benjamin H. Caballero, Robert J. Cousins, Katherine L. Tucker and Thomas R. Ziegler, (Lippincott Williams & Wilkins, eleventh edition, 2012), pp. 159–175.
24. Callum Livingstone, 'Review of copper provision in the parenteral nutrition of adults', *Nutrition in Clinical Practice*, 32:2 (2017), 153–165.
25. Luigi Ferrucci and Elisa Fabbri, 'Inflammageing: Chronic inflammation in ageing, cardiovascular disease, and frailty', *Nature Reviews Cardiology*, 15:9 (2018), 505–522.
26. A. Davidson and B. Diamond, 'Autoimmune diseases', *New England Journal of Medicine*, 345:5 (2001), 340–350.
27. Richard A. Festa and Dennis J. Thiele, 'Copper at the front line of the host-pathogen battle', *PLoS Pathogens*, 8:9 (2012).
28. Jacquelyn M. Powers and George R. Buchanan, 'Disorders of iron metabolism: New diagnostic and treatment approaches to iron

REFERENCES

deficiency', *Hematology/Oncology Clinics of North America*, 33:3 (2019), 393–408.
29. 'Iron', nhs.uk (3 August 2020).
30. N. R. Campbell, B. B. Hasinoff, H. Stalts, B. Rao and N. C. Wong, 'Ferrous sulfate reduces thyroxine efficacy in patients with hypothyroidism', *Annals of Internal Medicine*, 117:12 (1992), 1010–1013.

9. LOVE YOUR LIVER

1. Paul Kubes and Craig Jenne, 'Immune responses in the liver', *Annu Rev Immunol*, 26:36 (2018), 247–277.
2. Yavuz Emre Parlar, Sefika Nur Ayar, Deniz Cagdas and Yasemin H. Balaban, 'Liver immunity, autoimmunity, and inborn errors of immunity', *World Journal of Hepatology*, 15:1 (2023), 52–67.
3. K. Michael Pollard, Per Hultman and Dwight H. Kono, 'Toxicology of autoimmune diseases', *Chemical Research in Toxicology*, 23:3 (2010), 455–466.
4. Annarosa Floreani, Patrick S. C. Leung and M. Eric Gershwin, 'Environmental basis of autoimmunity', *Clinical Reviews in Allergy & Immunology*, 50:3 (2016), 287–300.
5. Christine G. Parks, Frederick W. Miller, Kenneth Michael Pollard, Carlo Selmi, Dori Germolec, Kelly Joyce, Noel R. Rose and Michael C. Humble, 'Expert panel workshop consensus statement on the role of the environment in the development of autoimmune disease', *Int J Mol Sci*, 15:8 (2014), 14269–14297.
6. Datis Kharrazian, 'Exposure to environmental toxins and autoimmune conditions', *Integrative Medicine (Encinitas)*, 20:2 (2021), 20–24.
7. Yony Román-Ochoa, Grethel Teresa Choque Delgado, Teresa R. Tejada, Harry R. Yucra, Antonio E. Durand and Bruce R. Hamaker, 'Heavy metal contamination and health risk assessment in grains and grain-based processed food in Arequipa region of Peru', *Chemosphere*, 274 (2021), 129792.
8. Sonia Collado-López, Larissa Betanzos-Robledo, Martha María Téllez-Rojo, Héctor Lamadrid-Figueroa, Moisés Reyes, Camilo Ríos and Alejandra Cantoral, 'Heavy metals in unprocessed or minimally processed foods consumed by humans worldwide: A scoping review', *International Journal of Environmental Research and Public Health*, 19:14 (2022), 8651.

9. K. P. Mishra, 'Lead exposure and its impact on immune system: A review', *Toxicology in Vitro*, 23:6 (2009), 969–972.
10. Priyanka Bist and Sangeeta Choudhary, 'Impact of heavy metal toxicity on the gut microbiota and its relationship with metabolites and future probiotics strategy: A review', *Biological Trace Element Research*, 200:12 (2022), 5328–5350.
11. 'Arsenic: general information', gov.uk (15 October 2024).
12. Khaled Ziani, Corina-Bianca Ioniță-Mîndrican, Magdalena Mititelu, Sorinel Marius Neacșu, Carolina Negrei, Elena Moroșan, Doina Drăgănescu and Olivia-Teodora Preda, 'Microplastics: A real global threat for environment and food safety: A state of the art review', *Nutrients*, 15:3 (2023), 617.
13. Qixiao Zhai, Arjan Narbad and Wei Chen, 'Dietary strategies for the treatment of cadmium and lead toxicity', *Nutrients*, 7:1 (2014), 552–571.
14. Y. Omura and S. L. Beckman, 'Role of mercury (Hg) in resistant infections & effective treatment of Chlamydia trachomatis and Herpes family viral infections (and potential treatment for cancer) by removing localized Hg deposits with Chinese parsley and delivering effective antibiotics using various drug uptake enhancement methods', *Acupuncture & Electro-Therapeutics Research*, 20:3–4 (1995), 195–229; Y. Omura, Y. Shimotsuura, A. Fukuoka, H. Fukuoka and T. Nomoto, 'Significant mercury deposits in internal organs following the removal of dental amalgam, & development of pre-cancer on the gingiva and the sides of the tongue and their represented organs as a result of inadvertent exposure to strong curing light (used to solidify synthetic dental filling material) & effective treatment: A clinical case report, along with organ representation areas for each tooth', *Acupunct Electrother Res*, 21:2 (1996), 133–160.
15. G. Park, H. G. Kim, Y. O. Kim, S. H. Park, S. Y. Kim and M. S. Oh, '*Coriandrum sativum L.* protects human keratinocytes from oxidative stress by regulating oxidative defense systems', *Skin Pharmacology and Physiology*, 25:2 (2012), 93–99.
16. Joseph Villarreal, Christopher A. Kahn, James V. Dunford, Ekta Patel and Richard F. Clark, 'A retrospective review of the prehospital use of activated charcoal', *American Journal of Emergency Medicine*, 33:1 (2015), 56–59.

REFERENCES

17. Shukry Zawdhir, Indika Gawarammana, Paul I. Dargan, Mahfoudh Abdulghni and Andrew H. Dawson, 'Activated charcoal significantly reduces the amount of colchicine released from Gloriosa superba in simulated gastric and intestinal media', *Clinical Toxicology (Philadelphia)*, 55:8 (2017), 914–918.
18. Jason Silberman, Michael A. Galuska and Alan Taylor, *Activated Charcoal* (StatPearls Publishing, 2023).
19. David N. Juurlink, 'Activated charcoal for acute overdose: A reappraisal', *British Journal of Clinical Pharmacology*, 81:3 (2016), 482–487.
20. Institute of Medicine, Food and Nutrition Board, *Dietary Reference Intakes for Water, Potassium, Sodium, Chloride, and Sulfate* (National Academy of Sciences Press, 2005); European Food Safety Authority, 'Scientific opinion on dietary reference values for water', *EFSA Journal*, 8:3 (2010), 1459–1507.
21. Roshan Patel and Matthew Mueller, *Alcohol-Associated Liver Disease* (StatPearls Publishing, 2023).

10. SORT YOUR MESS OUT!

1. Gregory E. Miller, Edith Chen, Jasmen Sze, Teresa Marin, Jesusa M. G. Arevalo, Richard Doll, Roy Ma and Steve W. Cole, 'A functional genomic fingerprint of chronic stress in humans: Blunted glucocorticoid and increased NF-kappaB signaling', *Biological Psychiatry*, 64:4 (2008), 266–272; Gregory E. Miller, Nicholas Rohleder and Steve W. Cole, 'Chronic interpersonal stress predicts activation of pro- and anti-inflammatory signaling pathways 6 months later', *Psychosomatic Medicine*, 71:1 (2009), 57–62; Michael R. Irwin and Steven W. Cole, 'Reciprocal regulation of the neural and innate immune systems', *Nat Rev Immunol*, 11:9 (2011), 625–632.
2. T. J. Strauman, A. M. Lemieux and C. L. Coe, 'Self-discrepancy and natural killer cell activity: Immunological consequences of negative self-evaluation', *Journal of Personality and Social Psychology*, 64:6 (1993), 1042–1052.
3. Robert Weiss, *Loneliness: The Experience of Emotional and Social Isolation* (The MIT Press, 1973).
4. *All in the Mind: The Loneliness Experiment*, BBC Radio 4 programme (2018).

5. 'Facts and statistics about loneliness', campaigntoendloneliness.org.
6. Ibid.
7. Simone Schnall, Kent D. Harber, Jeanine K. Stefanucci and Dennis R. Proffitt, 'Social support and the perception of geographical slant', *Journal of Experimental Social Psychology*, 44:5 (2008), 1246–1255.
8. Julianne Holt-Lunstad, Timothy B. Smith, Mark Baker, Tyler Harris and David Stephenson, 'Loneliness and social isolation as risk factors for mortality: A meta-analytic review', *Perspectives on Psychological Science*, 10:2 (2015), 227–237; Nicole K. Valtorta, Mona Kanaan, Simon Gilbody, Sara Ronzi and Barbara Hanratty, 'Loneliness and social isolation as risk factors for coronary heart disease and stroke: Systematic review and meta-analysis of longitudinal observational studies', *Heart*, 102:13 (2016), 1009–1016.
9. Robert S. Wilson, Kristin R. Krueger, Steven E. Arnold, Julie A. Schneider, Jeremiah F. Kelly, Lisa L. Barnes, Yuxiao Tang and David A. Bennett, 'Loneliness and risk of Alzheimer disease', *Archives of General Psychiatry*, 64:2 (2007), 234–240.
10. Homa Pourriyahi, Niloufar Yazdanpanah, Amene Saghazadeh and Nima Rezaei, 'Loneliness: An immunometabolic syndrome', *International Journal of Environmental Research and Public Health*, 18:22 (2021), 12162.
11. Michael R. Irwin and Steven W. Cole, 'Reciprocal regulation of the neural and innate immune systems', *Nat Rev Immunol*, 11:9 (2011), 625–632.
12. Gregory E. Miller, Edith Chen, Jasmen Sze, Teresa Marin, Jesusa M. G. Arevalo, Richard Doll, Roy Ma and Steve W. Cole, 'A functional genomic fingerprint of chronic stress in humans: Blunted glucocorticoid and increased NF-kappaB signaling', *Biol Psychiatry*, 64:4 (2008), 266–272.
13. Paul Grossman, Ludger Niemann, Stefan Schmidt and Harald Walach, 'Mindfulness-based stress reduction and health benefits. A meta-analysis', *Journal of Psychosomatic Research*, 57:1 (2004), 35–43; Roger Jahnke, Linda Larkey, Carol Rogers, Jennifer Etnier and Fang Lin, 'A comprehensive review of health benefits of qigong and tai chi', *American Journal of Health Promotion*, 24:6 (2010), e1–e25; Arndt

REFERENCES

Büssing, Thomas Ostermann, Rainer Lüdtke and Andreas Michalsen, 'Effects of yoga interventions on pain and pain-associated disability: A meta-analysis', *Journal of Pain*, 13:1 (2012), 1–9.

14. Martin E. P. Seligman, Tracy A. Steen, Nansook Park and Christopher Peterson, 'Positive psychology progress: Empirical validation of interventions', *American Psychologist*, 60:5 (2005), 410–421.

15. Fiona C. Bull, Salih S. Al-Ansari, Stuart Biddle, Katja Borodulin, Matthew P. Buman, Greet Cardon, Catherine Carty, Jean-Philippe Chaput, Sebastien Chastin, Roger Chou, Paddy C. Dempsey, Loretta DiPietro, Ulf Ekelund, Joseph Firth, Christine M. Friedenreich, Leandro Garcia, Muthoni Gichu, Russell Jago, Peter T. Katzmarzyk, Estelle Lambert, Michael Leitzmann, Karen Milton, Francisco B. Ortega, Chathuranga Ranasinghe, Emmanuel Stamatakis, Anne Tiedemann, Richard P. Troiano, Hidde P. van der Ploeg, Vicky Wari and Juana F. Willumsen, 'World Health Organization 2020 guidelines on physical activity and sedentary behaviour', *British Journal of Sports Medicine*, 54:24 (2020), 1451–1462.

16. David C. Nieman and Laurel M. Wentz, 'The compelling link between physical activity and the body's defense system', *Journal of Sport & Health Science*, 8:3 (2019), 201–217.

17. Ibid.

18. Ibid.

19. Zoltan Ungvari, Vince Fazekas-Pongor, Anna Csiszar and Setor K. Kunutsor, 'The multifaceted benefits of walking for healthy aging: From Blue Zones to molecular mechanisms', *GeroScience*, 45:6 (2023), 3211–3239.

20. Annina Seiler, Christopher P. Fagundes and Lisa M. Christian, *The Impact of Everyday Stressors on the Immune System and Health* (SpringerLink, 1970).

21. M. Herrmann, J. Schölmerich and R. H. Straub, 'Stress and rheumatic diseases', *Rheumatic Disease Clinics of North America*, 26:4 (2000), 737–763.

22. Hans Selye, 'A syndrome produced by diverse nocuous agents', *Nature*, 138:32 (1936).

23. Chenchen Wang, Raveendhara Bannuru, Judith Ramel, Bruce Kupelnick, Tammy Scott and Christopher H. Schmid, 'Tai chi on psychological well-being: Systematic review and meta-analysis', *BMC*

Complementary and Alternative Medicine, 10:23 (2010); Chenchen Wang, 'Role of tai chi in the treatment of rheumatologic diseases', *Current Rheumatology Reports*, 14:6 (2012), 598–603; Michael H. Antoni, Neil Schneiderman and Frank Penedo, 'Behavioural interventions: Immunologic mediators and disease outcomes', in *Psychoneuroimmunology, Volume 1*, ed. Robert Ader (Elsevier Academic Press, 2007), pp. 675–704.

24. Suzanne C. Segerstrom and Gregory E. Miller, 'Psychological stress and the human immune system: A meta-analytic study of 30 years of inquiry', *Psychological Bulletin*, 130:4 (2004), 601–630.
25. Haiyin Jiang, Zongxin Ling, Yonghua Zhang, Hongjin Mao, Zhanping Ma, Yan Yin, Weihong Wang, Wenxin Tang, Zhonglin Tan, Jianfei Shi, Lanjuan Li and Bing Ruan, 'Altered fecal microbiota composition in patients with major depressive disorder', *Brain, Behavior & Immunity*, 48 (2015), 186–194.
26. Guillaume Fond, Anderson Loundou, Nora Hamdani, Wahid Boukouaci, Aroldo Dargel, José Oliveira, Matthieu Roger, Ryad Tamouza, Marion Leboyer and Laurent Boyer, 'Anxiety and depression comorbidities in irritable bowel syndrome (IBS): A systematic review and meta-analysis', *European Archives of Psychiatry and Clinical Neuroscience*, 264:8 (2014), 651–660.
27. Janice K. Kiecolt-Glaser, Stephanie J. Wilson, Michael L. Bailey, Rebecca Andridge, Juan Peng, Lisa M. Jaremka, Christopher P. Fagundes, William B. Malarkey, Bryon Laskowsi and Martha A. Belury, 'Marital distress, depression, and a leaky gut: Translocation of bacterial endotoxin as a pathway to inflammation', *Psychoneuroendocrinology*, 98 (2018), 52–60.
28. Janice K. Kiecolt-Glaser, Diane L. Habash, Christopher P. Fagundes, Rebecca Andridge, Juan Peng, William B. Malarkey and Martha A. Belury, 'Daily stressors, past depression, and metabolic responses to high-fat meals: A novel path to obesity', *Biol Psychiatry*, 77:7 (2014), 653–660.
29. Jon Kabat-Zinn, *Wherever You Go, There You Are: Mindfulness Meditation in Everyday Life* (Hyperion Books, 1994).
30. David W. Orme-Johnson and Vernon A. Barnes, 'Effects of the transcendental meditation technique on trait anxiety: A meta-analysis of randomized controlled trials', *Journal of Alternative and Complementary Medicine*, 20:5 (2014), 330–341.

REFERENCES

31. David S. Black and George M. Slavich, 'Mindfulness meditation and the immune system: A systematic review of randomized controlled trials', *Annals of the New York Academy of Sciences*, 1373:1 (2016), 13–24.
32. Masoumeh Shohani, Gholamreza Badfar, Marzieh Parizad Nasirkandy, Sattar Kaikhavani, Shoboo Rahmati, Yaghoob Modmeli, Ali Soleymani and Milad Azami, 'The effect of yoga on stress, anxiety, and depression in women', *International Journal of Preventive Medicine*, 21:9 (2018), 21.
33. Chris C. Streeter, Theodore H. Whitfield, Liz Owen, Tasha Rein, Surya K. Karri, Aleksandra Yakhkind, Ruth Perlmutter, Andrew Prescot, Perry F. Renshaw, Domenic A. Ciraulo and J. Eric Jensen, 'Effects of yoga versus walking on mood, anxiety, and brain GABA levels: A randomized controlled MRS study', *Journal of Alternative and Complementary Medicine*, 16:11 (2010), 1145–1152.
34. U. Dalgas, E. Stenager and T. Ingemann-Hansen, 'Multiple sclerosis and physical exercise: Recommendations for the application of resistance-, endurance- and combined training', *Multiple Sclerosis*, 14:1 (2008), 35–53.
35. Nobuhiko Eda, Hironaga Ito and Takao Akama, 'Beneficial effects of yoga stretching on salivary stress hormones and parasympathetic nerve activity', *Journal of Sports Science and Medicine*, 19:4 (2020), 695–702.
36. Esther N. Moszeik, Timo von Oertzen and Karl-Heinz Renner, 'Effectiveness of a short yoga nidra meditation on stress, sleep, and well-being in a large and diverse sample', *Curr Psychol*, 41 (2022), 5272–5286.
37. Consensus Conference Panel, Nathaniel F. Watson, M. Safwan Badr, Gregory Belenky, Donald L. Bliwise, Orfeu M. Buxton, Daniel Buysse, David F. Dinges, James Gangwisch, Michael A. Grandner, Clete Kushida, Raman K. Malhotra, Jennifer L. Martin, Sanjay R. Patel, Stuart F. Quan and Esra Tasali, 'Recommended amount of sleep for a healthy adult: A joint consensus statement of the American Academy of Sleep Medicine and Sleep Research Society', *Sleep*, 38:6 (2015), 843–844.
38. Margot L. Zomers, Gerben Hulsegge, Sandra H. van Oostrom, Karin I. Proper, W. M. Monique Verschuren and H. Susan J. Picavet, 'Characterizing adult sleep behavior over 20 years: The population-based Doetinchem Cohort study', *Sleep*, 40:7 (2017).

39. Seithikurippu R. Pandi-Perumal, Asmaa M. Abumuamar, David Warren Spence, Vijay Kumar Chattu, Adam Moscovitch and Ahmed S. BaHammam, 'Racial/ethnic and social inequities in sleep medicine: The tip of the iceberg?', *Journal of the National Medical Association*, 109:4 (2017), 279–286.
40. J. Born, T. Lange, K. Hansen, M Mölle, and H. L. Fehm, 'Effects of sleep and circadian rhythm on human circulating immune cells', *Journal of Immunology*, 158:9 (1997), 4454–4464.
41. Kenneth D. Kochanek, Jiaquan Xu and Elizabeth Arias, *Mortality in the United States, 2019* (CDC, 2020), pp. 1–8.
42. Vivien C. Abad, Priscilla S. A. Sarinas and Christian Guilleminault, 'Sleep and rheumatologic disorders', *Sleep Medicine Reviews*, 12:3 (2008), 211–228.
43. 'Sleep problems', nhs.uk.
44. Christian Benedict, Heike Vogel, Wenke Jonas, Anni Woting, Michael Blaut, Annette Schürmann and Jonathan Cedernaes, 'Gut microbiota and glucometabolic alterations in response to recurrent partial sleep deprivation in normal-weight young individuals', *Molecular Metabolism*, 5:12 (2016), 1175–1186.
45. Yasmine Belkaid and Timothy W. Hand, 'Role of the microbiota in immunity and inflammation', *Cell*, 157:1 (2014), 121–141.
46. Eric Zhao, Christopher Tait, Carlod D. Minacapelli, Carolyn Catalano and Vinod K. Rustgi, 'Circadian rhythms, the gut microbiome, and metabolic disorders', *Gastro Hep Advances*, 1:1 (2022), 93–105.
47. Yuanyuan Li, Yanli Hao, Fang Fan and Bin Zhang, 'The role of microbiome in insomnia, circadian disturbance and depression', *Frontiers in Psychiatry*, 9 (2018), 669.
48. Christopher A. Thaiss, David Zeevi, Maayan Levy, Gili Zilberman-Schapira, Jotham Suez, Anouk C. Tengeler, Lior Abramson, Meirav N. Katz, Tal Korem, Niv Zmora, Yael Kuperman, Inbal Biton, Shlomit Gilad, Alon Harmelin, Hagit Shapiro, Zamir Halpern, Eran Segal and Eran Elinav, 'Transkingdom control of microbiota diurnal oscillations promotes metabolic homeostasis', *Cell*, 159:3 (2014), 514–529.
49. Amy C. Reynolds, Jessica L. Paterson, Sally A. Ferguson, Dragana Stanley, Kenneth P. Wright Jr. and Drew Dawson, 'The shift work and health research agenda: Considering changes in gut microbiota as a

pathway linking shift work, sleep loss and circadian misalignment, and metabolic disease', *Sleep Med Rev*, 34 (2017), 3–9.
50. JoEllen Wilbur, Arlene Michaels Miller, Judith McDevitt, Edward Wang and Josephine Miller, 'Menopausal status, moderate-intensity walking, and symptoms in midlife women', *Research and Theory for Nursing Practice*, 19:2 (2005), 163–180.
51. Moé Kishida and Steriani Elavsky, 'An intensive longitudinal examination of daily physical activity and sleep in midlife women', *Sleep Health*, 2:1 (2016), 42–48.
52. Alycia N. Sullivan Bisson, Stephanie A. Robinson and Margie E. Lachman, 'Walk to a better night of sleep: Testing the relationship between physical activity and sleep', *Sleep Health*, 5:5 (2019), 487–494.
53. Makoto Bannai and Nobuhiro Kawai, 'New therapeutic strategy for amino acid medicine: Glycine improves the quality of sleep', *J Pharmacol Sci*, 118:2 (2012), 145–148; Nobuhiro Kawai, Noriaki Sakai, Masashi Okuro, Sachie Karakawa, Yosuke Tsuneyoshi, Noriko Kawasaki, Tomoko Takeda, Makoto Bannai and Seiji Nishino, 'The sleep-promoting and hypothermic effects of glycine are mediated by NMDA receptors in the suprachiasmatic nucleus', *Neuropsychopharmacology*, 40:6 (2015), 1405–1416.

11. SHOULD I SUPPLEMENT?

1. Phoebe Tee Yon Ern, Tang Yin Quan, Fung Shin Yee and Adeline Chia Yoke Yin, 'Therapeutic properties of *Inonotus obliquus* (Chaga mushroom): A review', *Mycology*, 15:2 (2023), 144–161.
2. Su-Jin Jung, Eun-Soo Jung, Eun-Kyung Choi, Hong-Sig Sin, Ki-Chan Ha and Soo-Wan Chae, 'Immunomodulatory effects of a mycelium extract of Cordyceps (*Paecilomyces hepiali*; CBG-CS-2): A randomized and double-blind clinical trial', *BMC Complement Altern Med*, 19:1 (2019), 77.
3. R. K. Chandra, RETRACTED, 'Effect of vitamin and trace-element supplementation on immune responses and infection in elderly subjects', *Lancet*, 340:8828 (1992), 1124–1127.

Index

Page numbers in **bold** refer to tables.

adaptive immune system, overview of 17, 18–19
additives 59, 98, 104–5, 174, 214–20
adenoids 16
ADHD (Attention Deficit Hyperactivity Disorder) 217
adipose tissue *see* fat, body
adrenaline 98
advanced glycaemic end products (AGEs) 68
ageing
   and allergies 49, 52, 53
   and autoimmune disease 2, 27, 28, 36, 41, 44–5
   and blood-sugar levels 68, 69
   and gum disease 86
   hormonal fluctuations 2, 41
   immunosenescence 44–5, 189, 190, 193
   loss of muscle mass 99, 123
   managing via exercise 189, 190, 192, 193–4
   managing via supplements 229
   and nutritional deficiencies 136–7, 138, 151–2, 155
   reduced lymphocyte production 13, 16, 45, 190
   shrinkage of adenoids 16
   shrinkage of thymus 16, 45, 190
   and stress management 196
alcohol 88, 97, 103–4, 116, 140, 178
algae supplements 128
allergies
   and ageing 52, 53
   antibody overresponses 47
   asthma 53–5
   atopic march 48
   eczema 48–50
   food allergies *see* food allergies
   gender differences 52, 53
   and genetics 48, 50, 52, 54
   and gut microbiome 47–8, 57, 60
   hay fever 51–3
   and heavy metals toxicity 166
   hygiene hypothesis 78
   maternal diet impacts on child 54–5, 56–8
   and obesity 53
   and oral microbiome 86
   rise in 47–8, 65
   types 47

INDEX

alpha-linolenic acid (ALA) 127, 223;
    see also omega-3 fatty acids
alpha lipoic acid (ALA), 175–6
Alzheimer's disease 20, 86, 138, 184,
    223–4
amino acids 101, 120–1, 123, 165, 174,
    175, 189, 209–10, 228
anaemia 30, 31, 138–9, 140–1, 158, 159
anti-inflammatory compounds
    amino acids 101, 123
    butyrate 102, 111
    carbohydrates 192
    carotenoids 118
    in fibre 102, 109–10, 111
    micronutrients 131, 132, 141, 142,
        145, 146, 149, 151, 153, 154
    monounsaturated fats
        (MUFAs) 128
    myconutrients 119, 120, 227
    polyphenols 100, 101, 103–4,
        116–18
    polyunsaturated fats 126–7, 137,
        174, 223–4
    prebiotics 102
    probiotics 225
    sex hormones 41
antibiotics 61, 65, 78, 79, 81, 150
antibodies
    and allergies 47, 59
    and autoimmune disease 27, 29, 33
    defining 12
    IgE antibodies 59
    loneliness impacts 185
    nutritional requirements 120, 122,
        135, 151, 152
    probiotic impacts 225

antigens 12, 18
antioxidants
    carbohydrates 109
    carotenoids 118
    fighting oxidative stress 67, 116
    glutathione 153, 165, 174, 175–6
    lipoic acid (ALA) 175–6
    myconutrients 119, 120, 226, 227
    polyphenols 100, 101, 103–4,
        116–18
    toxins as risk to 165
    vitamins and minerals 131, 132, 145,
        151, 152–3, 174
arginine 123
arsenic 163, 167, 169–71; see also
    heavy metals
arthritis, rheumatoid (RA) see
    rheumatoid arthritis (RA)
Asparagus and Mozzarella Salad
    259–60
aspartame 70–1
asthma 48, 49, 53–5, 86, 217
atherosclerosis 21, 222
atopic march 48
autoimmune disease; see also
    allergies; specific disease
    and ageing 27, 28, 36
    and body part affected 25
    as cause of mortality 26
    defining 24
    diagnosis, importance of
        early 26
    mosaic of autoimmunity 25–6
    multiple autoimmune syndrome
        (MAS) 26
    numbers of 24

INDEX

nutritional treatments 127, 135, 140, 149
polyautoimmunity 26
rise in 1, 24, 25
risk factors
  ageing 2, 28, 41, 44–5
  diet 30, 43–4, 72, 98, 104
  gender 2, 25, 27, 29, 32, 37, 40–2, 64
  genetics 2, 25, 26, 27, 32, 34, 36, 37, 39–40, 164
  gut microbiome health, poor 25, 26, 44, 71, 77, 80, 81–2, 141–2
  hormonal fluctuations 27, 29, 40–2
  infections 32, 34, 37, 45
  lectin 97
  nutritional deficiencies 138–40, 141, 146, 153, 155
  oral microbiome health, poor 85
  smoking 32
  stress 42–3
  toxins 163, 164–5, 166–7, 168, 169, 171

B cells 12–13, 18, 41, 84
bacteria, bad *see* infections
bacteria, good *see* gut microbiome; oral microbiome
Bacteroides spp. 104, 207–8
balance, immune system 3, 13, 17, 19, 79, 93
Beet It Burgers 286–7
beta-carotene 118, 147, 148
beta-glucans 110, 119
Bifidobacteria spp. 60, 83, 225

bioaccumulation 168
bioavailability, definition of 213–14
blood cholesterol levels 125
blood clotting 126, 148–9
blood sugar levels 44, 68–71, 73, 75, 108–9, 112, 125
Blue Zones 193–4
body composition 72–5
body mass index (BMI) 43, 73–4
bone health 31, 85, 132, 142–3, 148, 150, 230; *see also* rheumatoid arthritis (RA)
bone marrow 12, 14, 15
brain health; *see also* mental health
  cerebrovascular disease 192
  dementia 20
  gut–brain communication 76–7, 81, 196–7, 223–4
  multiple sclerosis (MS) 31–3
  protection factors
    blood–brain barrier 20, 165, 172
    glycine intake 210
    healthy gut microbiome 76–7, 102
    healthy mitochondria 67
    microglia 20
    myconutrient intake 226
    omega-3 fatty acid intake 223–4
    physical activity and exercise 192
    sleep/rest 178–9, 209
    sunlight exposure 209
  risk factors
    dysbiosis 81, 196
    genetics 20
    gluten 30

INDEX

brain health – cont'd.
    gum disease 86
    immune malfunction 20
    inflammation 20
    loneliness 184–5
    stress *see* stress
    toxins 165, 166, 167–8, 172
    vitamin B deficiencies 138
breastfeeding 40, 57, 134
breathing exercises 204
Brunch Bruschetta 249–50
butyrate 102, 111, 190, 191, 207

cadmium 167; *see also* heavy metals
caffeine 59, 97, 98, 101, 210–11
calcium 142, 144, 230
calorie intake 43, 73, 107, 129, **232**
cancer
    and infection risk 64
    protection factors 102, 112, 116, 119, 120, 133, 145, 188, 227
    risk factors 13, 22, 26, 72, 75, 85, 87, 88, 124, 125, 190, 206; *see also* carcinogens
    surveillance and responses to 1, 11, 12, 13, 161
carbohydrates 58, 59–60, 69–70, 97, 99–100, 107–9, 111, 115–20, 192, **232**; *see also* fibre
carcinogens 167, 170, 215–16, 217, 218–19
cardiovascular health *see* heart and arteries health
carotenoids 118, 147
carrageenan 218
cereals; *see also* grains, whole

alpha-lipoic acid (ALA) 176
carbohydrates 108
cysteine 175
fibre 57, 58, 110
food allergens 56, 174
fructans 60
micronutrients 124, 142, 144, 145, 156, 158, **233**, **234**
prebiotics **103**
refined grains 97, 108, 155
toxins 166
charcoal, activated 176–8
chemicals, dietary *see* additives
Chicken and Chickpea Curry 280–1
Chilli Pepper Cod 282–3
chocolate **103**, 117, 156, 167, 210–11, 222, **233**
cholesterol 125, 126, 218
circadian rhythm 207–9
Clostridiales spp. 104, 207–8
Clostridioides difficile 84
coeliac disease 30–1, 140, 146, 150, 153, 155, 156–7
coffee 97, 98, 101, 117, 158
collagen 123, 209–10, 228
colourings, artificial 218–19
constipation 34, 59, 80, 82, 84, 113, 159, 177
copper 156–7, 214, **233**
cortisol 98, 189, 194–5, 197, 200, 201, 227
Covid-19 *see* SARS-CoV-2 virus (Covid-19)
Creamy Vegetable Red Curry 269–70
Crohn's disease 127, 140, 146, 155, 217

cysteine 165, 175
cystic fibrosis 150
cytokines 40, 84, 135, 138, 151, 154, 172, 197, 225

daily intake recommendations
    fat 129
    fibre 112, 114
    minerals 152, 153–4, 155, 157, 158–9
    protein 99, 122–3
    table **232–4**
    vitamins 133–4, 135–6, 137, 143, 145, 147, 149
    water 64, 177
dairy products 97, 101, 121, 139, 144, 147, 152, 158, 171
deficiencies, nutritional 63, 72, 160, 214
    minerals 31, 132, 151–2, 153, 154, 155, 156–7, 158–9, 222
    omega-3 fatty acids 223–4
    protein 122
    supplements for *see* supplements, nutritional
    vitamins 47, 136–7, 138–41, 142, 144, 146, 150, 175, 221
dementia 20, 138, 184, 192
dental check-ups 88
depression 138, 148, 187, 195, 196, 197–8, 199, 201, 206
detoxification programme 173–9
diabetes, type 1 25, 35–6, 80, 141
diabetes, type 2
    defining 36
    risk factors 21, 22, 70–1, 85, 124, 155, 179, 206, 207, 218, 222

    risk prevention 111, 188, 192, 210
disaccharides 108–9, 111
diversity, diet 56–7, 58, 76, 78, 99–100, 106, 118, 130, 131, 160, 173–4, 179, 213
docosahexaenoic acid (DHA) 127, 223, 224; *see also* omega-3 fatty acids
dysbiosis 26, 44, 70, 80–1, 85, 93–5, 105, 167, 196, 206–7

eczema (atopic dermatitis) 48–50, 53
eggs 50, 56, 98, 121, 124, 144, 147, 158, 174, **232–4**
eicosapentaenoic acid (EPA) 127, 223, 224; *see also* omega-3 fatty acids
emulsifiers 98, 104–5; *see also* additives
endocrine system 73, 166, 206; *see also* hormones; *specific gland*
endorphins 200
Enterococcus faecalis 104
epigenetics 39
Epstein–Barr virus 32, 45
ergosterol 120, 144
Escherichia coli 217
exercise *see* physical activity and exercise
eye health 31, 37–8, 51, 146

Fabulous Frittata 257–8
faecal microbiota transplantation (FMT) 83–4
Faecalibacterium spp. 83
fat, body 72–5, 166

INDEX

fat (in diet) 99, 113, 125–30, 144, 145, 148, 149, 218, **232**; *see also* omega-3 fatty acids
fat-malabsorption disorders 146, 150, 155
fermented foods 78, 101–2, 213, 224, 225, **234**
fever 62–3, 66–7
fibre
    and allergies 57–8
    and blood-sugar levels 69–70, 108
    content in common foods 114
    deficiency and mortality rates 113
    health benefits 111–12, 113
    insoluble 58, 110
    and iron absorption 158
    prebiotic 58, 102, **103**, 110, 119
    recommended daily intake 112, 114, **232**
    removing and reintroducing 97, 102
    resistant starch 58, 111
    soluble 57, 109–10
    tips for intake 115
fish; *see also* salmon; seafood
    food allergen 50, 56, 57, 174
    omega-3 fatty acids 127, 128, 223, 224, **234**
    protein 101, 121, 125, **232**
    toxins 166, 168, 170
    vitamins and minerals 124, 139, 144, 147, 149, **233**, **234**
flavourings, artificial 218–19; *see also* additives
FODMAP foods 110, 111
food allergies

additives 216, 217, 218
antigens 12
and detoxification 174
and eczema 50
versus food intolerances 59–60
IgE food allergies 59
major allergens 56
maternal diet impacts on child 54–5, 56–8
and oral microbiome 86
rise in 56
food intolerance 59–60, 98
food table **232–4**
fortified foods 124, 136, 142, 144, **233**, **234**
free radicals 115, 116, 117–18, 145, 153, 159, 165, 215, 217; *see also* oxidative stress
fructans 59–60
Fruit and Nut Chocolate 298–9
fruits and vegetables; *see also* legumes
    carbohydrates 108, **232**
    cysteine 175
    diversity of 99–100, 160
    edible peel 115
    fibre 57–8, 97, 110, 111, **232**
    five-a-day recommendation 133–4
    fructans 60
    glutamine 101
    healthy fats 99, 128
    lipoic acid (ALA) 176
    micronutrients 174
    phytonutrients 116, 117, 118
    prebiotics **103**, **234**
    sugars **233**

toxins 166
vitamins and minerals 132, 133, 145, 147, 149, 155, 158, 174, 213, 222, **233**, **234**
Fusobacterium nucleatum 87

garlic 58, 100, **103**, 110, 174, 175, **234**
gastrointestinal health; *see also specific disease/condition*
   additives impacts 104, 217, 218
   alcohol impacts 104
   enteric nervous system 208
   FODMAP foods 111
   and nutritional deficiencies 140, 155, 222
   oral microbiome impacts 86–7
   stress impacts 197
   toxin impacts 165, 166
genetics
   and allergies 48, 50, 52, 54
   and autoimmune disease 2, 25, 26, 27, 32, 34, 36, 37, 39–40, 164
   concordance 52
   and dementia 20
   epigenetics 39
   and food intolerances 98
   gene–environment interactions 55, 164
   genotoxicity 215
   and glutathione levels 175
   GWAS 54
   HLA genes 18, 39
   and immune response to pathogens 62
gingivitis 85, 86
glandular fever 32, 45

glucocorticoids 195
glucose (in blood) *see* blood sugar levels
glucose intolerance 70, 218
glutamate 165, 175
glutamine 101, 123
glutathione 153, 165, 174, 175–6
gluten 30, 56, 97, 100
glycine 165, 175, 209–10, 228
Good Gut Health Plan
   additives, avoiding 104–5
   alcohol 103–4
   journalling 96
   stage 1 – foods to remove 96–8
   stage 1 – foods to include 98–100
   stage 2 – reintroducing foods 100–2, **103**
grains, refined 97, 108, 155
grains, whole; *see also* cereals
   and blood-sugar levels 69
   carbohydrates 108, **232**
   fibre 58, 113, **232**
   minerals 152, 155, 156, **234**
   phytonutrients 116, 118
   protein 121, 125
   reintroducing 100
gratitude journalling 186–7
Green Lentil Soup 255–6
Guillain–Barré syndrome 45
gut-associated lymphoid tissue (GALT) 77–8
gut, leaky *see* leaky gut syndrome
gut microbiome
   and allergies 47–8, 57, 58, 60
   and autoimmune disease 25, 26, 44, 77

INDEX

gut microbiome – *cont'd.*
  description 76
  dysbiosis (imbalance) *see* dysbiosis
  faecal microbiota transplantation
    (FMT) 83–4
  functions 76–7
  gut–brain communication 76–7, 81,
    196–7, 223–4
  leaky gut syndrome *see* leaky gut
    syndrome
  link with immune system 22, 76,
    77–8, 79, 80, 88
  'microbes' defined 76, 78, 88–9
  promotion factors; *see also* Good
    Gut Health Plan
    beta-glucans 119
    carbohydrates 69
    diet diversity 78, 160
    exercise 190–1
    fibre 58, 60, 110, 113
    omega-3 fatty acids 223–4
    polyphenols 100, 103–4, 117
    prebiotics 58, 60, **103**, 110
    probiotics 83, 213, 224–5
    resistant starch 111
    vitamins 137, 142, 150
  protein production 122
  risk factors
    additives 70, 104–5, 217, 219
    antibiotics 79, 150
    high fat intake 126
    hormone imbalance 42, 197
    inactive lifestyle 191
    poor diet 44, 80–1
    sleep deprivation 206–7, 208
    stress 196–7

  toxins 167, 172
  ultra-processed foods 78–9
  vitamin D deficiency 141
  and sleep 206–8
  training/educating 78, 79
  vitamin K production 150

haemoglobin 14, 139, 157, 158
Hashimoto's disease 33–5, 154
hay fever (allergic rhinitis) 48, 51–3
heart and arteries health
  protection factors
    balance of omega-6:omega-3
     fatty acids 127
    fibre intake 102, 111, 113
    glycine intake 209–10
    healthy fat intake 126, 128–9
    immune system support 21–2
    physical activity and exercise
     188, 192, 200, 203
    sleep/rest 179
    vitamin A intake 146
    vitamin C intake 133
  risk factors
    artificial sweeteners 71
    atherosclerosis 21, 222
    autoimmune disease 25, 26
    chronic inflammation 22
    copper deficiency 156
    high blood cholesterol 125
    hyper-immune responses 62
    inflammation 20
    loneliness 184, 185
    meat intake 124, 125
    sleep deprivation 205, 206
    stress 195

INDEX

toxins 166, 167
trans fat intake 218
unhealthy oral microbiome 85, 86
vitamin B deficiencies 139
vitamin D toxicity 144
and susceptibility to infections 64
heavy metals 163, 166–71, 172, 173–6, 177
herbs and spices 100, 118, 174, 176, 213
hormones
additive impacts 217
age-related fluctuations 2, 230
and autoimmune disease 29, 33, 34–5, 40–2
and blood-sugar levels 68–9
exercise benefits 190, 192, 200, 201
and immune response to pathogens 61
insulin 35–6, 68, 69
iron requirement 157
melatonin 209
production by body fat 73, 125
production by gut microbiome 77
sex hormones 2, 29, 40–2, 230
stress hormones 98, 189, 194–5, 197, 200
thyroid hormones 33, 34–5, 153
human leucocyte antigen (HLA) immunity genes 18, 39
hydration 64, 177
hydrogenated oils 113, 129–30, 218
hygiene 38, 64, 78, 81, 85, 87–8
hyperthyroidism 34
hypothalamic–pituitary–adrenal (HPA) axis 195–6
hypothyroidism 33, 34, 35, 160

IgE food allergies 59–60
immune dysregulation 43, 60, 138, 145, 164, 165, 166, 189
immune modulation 17
immune tolerance 162
immunoglobulins 59, 225
immunological memory 18–19
immunometabolism 21, 44, 66–75, 80, 81, 113
immunosenescence 44–5, 189
immunosuppression 166, 170–1, 195
infections
and autoimmune disease 45, 81–2
definition and overview 60–1
economic impacts 63
and gut microbiome health 80, 84, 222, 225
immunological memory 19
and oral microbiome health 84–5, 86
protection factors
adequate rest/sleep 64–5
body's own defences 12–13, 14–19, 67, 84, 153, 161, 181–2
exercise 188, 189
hydration 64
hygiene 64
macronutrients 101, 107, 109–10, 117–18, 119, 120, 128, 226, 227
micronutrients 131–2, 135, 141, 142, 147, 153, 156, 157, 222, 229
sunlight 144
vaccines 60, 64
risk factors
ageing 193
gender 40, 61
inactive lifestyle 190

339

INDEX

infections – *cont'd.*
    individual differences 61–3
    liver damage 162, 163
    loneliness 185
    mineral deficiencies 151, 152, 154, 156, 157
    negative self-evaluation 181
    obesity 72
    protein deficiency 122
    sleep deprivation 205–6
    stress 194–5
    toxins 165, 170
    unhealthy oral microbiome 84–5, 86
    vitamin D deficiency 141
  typical annual number in adults 64
inflammasome 67
inflammation; *see also* anti-inflammatory compounds
  acute versus chronic 21–2
  and autoimmune disease *see* autoimmune disease
  cytokines 40, 84, 135
  reduction strategies 185–6, 188, 196, 199; *see also* anti-inflammatory compounds
  triggers
    additives 104
    ageing 44–5
    alcohol 104
    blood-sugar roller coaster 68
    damaged mitochondria 67
    decreased oestrogen levels 2, 41
    dysbiosis 81, 105
    gum disease 85–6
    high-carb meals 108
    immune imbalance 17
    inactive lifestyle 190
    intense physical activity 191–2
    leaky gut syndrome 105
    metabolic disturbances 20–1
    nutritional deficiencies 135, 140, 151, 153, 154, 156, 222
    overnutrition 72, 73, 107
    sleep deprivation 205, 206, 207
    stress 181, 185, 195, 197
    toxins 159, 164, 165, 172, 215, 217, 218
    ultra-processed foods 43, 44, 72
    unbalanced omega-6:omega-3 intake 127–8
    unhealthy fats 128–9, 129–30
inflammatory bowel diseases 85, 87, 195, 223; *see also* Crohn's disease
innate immune system, overview of 17–18
insulin 35–6, 68, 69, 155, 197–8, 207
interferon system 61
inulin 110
iodine 35, 229
iron 31, 132, 157–60, 214, **234**
irritable bowel syndrome (IBS) 60, 197, 218

kidney health 155, 166, 222

Lactobacilli spp. 60, 83, 100, 104, 197, 207–8, 225
lauric acid 99
lead 167; *see also* heavy metals

leaky gut syndrome 44, 77, 81–4, 93, 95–6, 99, 105, 141, 197
legumes 58, 69, 97, 101, **103**, 111, 113, 121, 123, 125, 155, 160, 222, **232**, **234**
Lemon and Blueberry Pancakes 290–1
Lemongrass Salmon 276–7
leptin 217
leucine 121
liver 15, 104, 148, 161–3, 165, 166, 174, 177, 178, 179, 210
loneliness 182–5, 212
lungs *see* respiratory health
lupus 29–30, 37, 127, 141, 195
lymph 14, 15, 64, 190, 203
lymph nodes 13, 14–15
lymphatic system 14–16
lymphatic vessels 14–15, 222
lymphocytes 12–13, 18, 38, 41, 47, 58, 84, 142, 170; *see also* natural killer (NK) cells; T cells

macronutrients 106–7, 130, 213; *see also specific macronutrient*
macrophages 47, 62, 161, 170, 189
magnesium 154–6, 214, 216, 222, **234**
magnesium stearate 216
maltodextrin 217
manganese 61
meats
   organ (offal) 147, 153, 156, 176, **233**, **234**
   poultry 101, 121, 123, 129, 139, 152, 175, **232**, **233**, **234**
   red 121, 124–5, 139, 152, 157, 158–9, 176, **232**, **233**, **234**
meditation 185–6, 198–9, 201–2
medium-chain fatty acids (MCFAs) 99

melatonin 209
mental health
   protection strategies 185–7, 192, 196, 198–204
   risk factors 25, 138, 148, 181–5, 206; *see also* stress
mercury 168–9, 175; *see also* heavy metals
metabolic homeostasis 21
metabolic syndrome 67, 70, 113, 127, 134, 184, 185
metabolism
   circadian rhythm disruption impacts 207
   defining 20, 66
   fibre, benefits of 112
   and gut microbiome health 69–70, 76, 80, 81, 113
   immunometabolism 21, 44, 66–75, 80, 81, 113
   liver's detoxification role 163
   loneliness impacts 184, 185
   metabolic homeostasis 21
   micronutrient requirements 132, 145, 157
   omega-6:omega-3 ratio 127
   stress impacts 197–8
   thyroid hormones impacts 34
   toxin impacts 172
   type 2 diabetes *see* diabetes, type 2
methylmercury 168
microbes *see* gut microbiome; oral microbiome
microglia 20
micronutrients 131, 160, 213, 214, 231; *see also specific vitamin, mineral*

INDEX

microplastics 171–3
mind–body therapies 185–6, 196
mindfulness 186, 198, 199, 201, 204
minerals *see specific mineral*
Miso Aubergines 263–4
mitochondria 66–7
Mixed Berry Porridge 239–40
monosaccharides 108–9, 111
mosaic of autoimmunity 25–6
multiple sclerosis (MS) 31–3, 81, 141, 195
muscle health 72, 73–4, 99, 123, 189; *see also* physical activity and exercise; *specific condition/illness*
myconutrients (mushrooms) 119–20, 144, 226–7
myeloid cells 62
myoglobin 157

natural killer (NK) cells 13, 120, 142, 161, 181–2, 192, 199, 206, 227
nervous system health
  enteric nervous system 208
  multiple sclerosis (MS) 31–3
  promotion factors 76, 126
  protection factors 201
  risk factors 136–7, 138, 139, 166, 169, 181, 195, 208
  sympathetic nervous system 182, 195
neutrophils 12, 14
noradrenaline 195
nuts and seeds
  carbohydrates 69
  fibre 57, 58, 113
  food allergens 50, 56, 174

healthy fats 99, 127, 128, 174, **232**
micronutrients 145, 149, 152, 153, 155, 156, 158, 222, **233**, **234**
prebiotics **103**, **234**
protein 98, 121, 122, 125, **232**

obesity 20, 21, 43, 44, 53, 70, 71–2, 75, 134, 207
oestrogen 2, 29, 41, 61, 230
oils 99, 118, 126, 127, 128, 129, 145, 147, 149, 216, 218, **232**, **233**
omega-3 fatty acids 57, 63, 126–8, 174, 223–4, 229, **234**
omega-6 fatty acids 126–8
optic neuritis 31
oral microbiome 84–8, 89
osteomalacia 143
Overnight Fruit and Nut Oats 243–4
overnutrition 72, 107, 138
oxidative stress 24, 67, 108, 116, 151, 164, 165, 172, 192, 222
oxycytosis 14

pancreas 35–6, 69
Parkinson's disease 80
pathogens *see* infections
Peanut Butter and Hazelnut Cookies 292–3
peanuts 50, 56, 174, **233**
Pecan and Date Balls 294–5
Pecan Protein Pancakes 241–2
Peplau, Hildegard 182
perimenopause 2, 41, 230
periodontitis 85–6
phagocytes 18, 162
phosphate 142

342

INDEX

physical activity and exercise
   balance 191
   and blood-sugar levels 69
   and carbohydrate intake 192
   dangers of intense activity 191–2
   defining 187–8
   health benefits 188, 192, 193
   improving sleep 209
   mind–body therapies 185–6
   and protein intake 99
   recommended weekly amount 188–9, **235**
   regularity and frequency 192
   role in lymph circulation 15
   as stress-management technique 200–4
   walking 192–4
phytic acid 100
phytonutrients 97, 115–20, 213
polyautoimmunity 26
polyphenols 100, 101, 103–4, 116–18
Potato, Spinach and Chickpea Stew 284–5
prebiotics 58, 60, 102–3, **103**, 110, 119, **234**
pregnancy
   and allergies 54–5, 57, 58–9
   and autoimmune disease 2, 34, 35, 38–9, 41
   and maternal diet 35, 54–5, 57, 58–9, 134, 136, 148, 151, 176, 229–30, **233**, **234**
   and smoking 54
preservatives 98, 104–5, 124, 217; *see also* additives
probiotics 83, 101–2, 213, 224–5, **234**

progesterone 41
protein (in diet) 71, 97, 98–9, 120–5, **232**; *see also* fish; legumes; meats; seafood
psoriasis 127, 223

qigong 185–6
questionnaires 4–7, 93–5, 95–6

Raspberry and Almond Pot 245–6
recipes
   breakfast
      Mixed Berry Porridge 239–40
      Overnight Fruit and Nut Oats 243–4
      Pecan Protein Pancakes 241–2
      Raspberry and Almond Pot 245–6
      Sliced Nutty Apple 247–8
   dinner
      Beet It Burgers 286–7
      Chicken and Chickpea Curry 280–1
      Chilli Pepper Cod 282–3
      Creamy Vegetable Red Curry 269–70
      Lemongrass Salmon 276–7
      Potato, Spinach and Chickpea Stew 284–5
      Stir-Fried Chinese Tofu 278–9
      Tofu Pumpkin Curry 288–9
      Turkey and Butternut Squash Lasagne 271–3
      Veggie Biryani 274–5
   lunch
      Asparagus and Mozzarella Salad 259–60
      Brunch Bruschetta 249–50

343

INDEX

recipes – *cont'd.*
    Fabulous Frittata 257–8
    Green Lentil Soup 255–6
    Miso Aubergines 263–4
    Stuffed Portobello Mushrooms 251–2
    Tofu Butternut Burgers 267–8
    Ultimate Stir-Fry 265–6
    Wild Rice Salad 261–2
    Zesty Spinach Soup 253–4
  sweet treats
    Fruit and Nut Chocolate 298–9
    Lemon and Blueberry Pancakes 290–1
    Peanut Butter and Hazelnut Cookies 292–3
    Pecan and Date Balls 294–5
    Warm Cinnamon Apple Pudding 296–7
recommended daily intake **232–4**
red blood cells (erythrocytes) 14, 135, 136, 137, 139, 157, 158
respiratory health 63–4, 84–5, 147, 153, 167, 189; *see also specific condition/illness*
rheumatoid arthritis (RA) 27–8, 81, 85, 87, 127, 135, 195, 223
rhinovirus (common cold) 19, 132, 152
rhodopsin 146
rickets 142
Roseburia spp. 83

Saccharomyces spp. 83, 225
salmon 98, 125, 127, 128, 144, 168, 223, **232–4**
Salmonella spp. 217

salt 125, 216, **233**
Sanskrit 200
SARS-CoV-2 virus (Covid-19) 18, 19, 45, 61, 62, 80, 132, 193
seafood 128, 153, 157, **233**; *see also* fish; shellfish
seeds *see* nuts and seeds
selenium 57, 152–4, **234**
Selye, Hans 195
shellfish 12, 56, 97, 152, 156, 168, 174, **232–4**; *see also* seafood
short-chain fatty acids (SCFAs) 60, 77, 102, 110, 111, 137, 190, 207
Sjögren, Henrik 37
Sjögren's syndrome 2, 37–9
sleep 63, 102, 132–3, 178–9, 205–11, 228, **235**
Sliced Nutty Apple 247–8
smoking 52–3, 54, 88, 116, 134, 170
sodium benzoate 217
sodium nitrite 104
spices *see* herbs and spices
spleen 15, 172
Stir-Fried Chinese Tofu 278–9
stress
  and autoimmune disease 28, 34, 42–3, 194
  conflicting roles on immune system 195
  and depression 197–8
  hormones 98, 189, 194–5, 197, 200, 201, 227
  HPA axis 195–6
  impacts on gut microbiome 196–7
  impacts on immune system 194–5, 196

impacts on metabolism 197–8
impacts on sleep 208
and NK cells 182
stress management
   gratitude journalling 186–7
   mind–body therapies 185–6, 196, 198–204
   mushrooms 227
   social connections 184
   supplements 123, 228–9
Stuffed Portobello Mushrooms 251–2
sugar (in diet) 43, 54, 70, 81, 88, 97, 108–9, 112, 113, **233**
Sullivan, Harry Stack 182
sulphur 174, 175
sunlight 63, 141, 142, 143–4, 208–9, 221, 231, **235**
supplements, nutritional
   additives to avoid 214–19
   balance 214
   collagen 228
   dangers 135–6, 136–7, 144, 146, 148, 150, 156, 159–60, 214–19, 221
   glycine 209–10, 228
   medication interactions 140, 142, 146, 148, 160, 210, 220, 226, 230
   minerals 35, 152, 153, 154, 155–6, 156–7, 159–60, 216, 222, 229
   myconutrients 119–20, 144, 226–7
   omega-3 fatty acids 128, 223–4, 229
   probiotics 102, 224–5
   reading labels 214–20
   unnecessary in diverse diet 213–14

vitamins 132, 134, 135–6, 137–8, 142–3, 144, 146, 148, 150, 221, 228–9, 230
surveillance, immune 11, 13, 14, 15, 18, 64, 181–2
sweeteners, artificial 59, 70–1, 98, 219; *see also* additives

T cells
   age impacts on production 13, 16, 45, 190
   excessive production of 81–2
   exercise benefits 189, 190
   meditation benefits 199
   microbiome impacts 77, 84, 151
   nutritional requirements for 135, 142, 144
   role 18
   sex hormone impacts 41
   toxin impacts 164
tai chi 185–6
talc 219
testosterone 41, 61
thymus 12, 16, 45, 146–7, 151, 172, 190
thyroid 30, 33–5, 153, 160, 169
titanium dioxide 215–16
Tofu Butternut Burgers 267–8
Tofu Pumpkin Curry 288–9
tonsils 16
toxins
   and autoimmune disease 163–4, 164–5, 166–7, 168, 169, 171
   body's defences against 14, 77, 161, 163
   defining 163
   detoxification 173–9

INDEX

toxins – *cont'd.*
   examples 163–4
   heavy metals 166–71, 172
   microplastics 171–3
   titanium dioxide 215–16
   toxic load 165
   and vitamin deficiencies 175
   vitamin/mineral toxicities 135–6, 144, 146, 148, 150, 156, 159–60, 176, 214, 221, 230, 231
Tregs (regulatory T cells) 13, 41, 58, 142
Turkey and Butternut Squash Lasagne 271–3

ulcerative colitis 83, 84, 127, 150
Ultimate Stir-Fry 265–6
ultra-processed foods 43–4, 78, 113, 127, 129–30, 140, 173, 174
ultraviolet (UV) light 143, 144, 221, 231

vaccines 19, 60, 64, 185, 186
vegan/vegetarian diet 97, 121, 125, 137–8, 139–40, 158, 214, 216, 229
vegetables *see* fruits and vegetables
Veggie Biryani 274–5
vinegar 71
viruses 61; *see also* infections; *specific virus*
vitamins
   A 146–8, 176, 221, 230, 231, **233**
   B complex 134–5, 214, 221
   B1 175
   B6 (pyridoxine) 135–6, 175, **233**
   B9 (folic acid/folate) 136–7, 138, 139, 140–1, 229, 231, **233**
   B12 (cobalamin) 124, 137–41, 214, 229, **233**
   C 61, 131–4, 158, 174, 175, 214, 217, 221, 228–9, 231, **233**
   D 120, 141–4, 154, 209, 221, 229, 230, 231, **233**
   E 54–5, 145–6, 221, 231, **233**
   K 148–50, 214, 221, **233**
   multivitamin supplements 229
   toxicities 135–6, 144, 146, 148, 176, 221, 230, 231

waist-to-height ratio (WHtR) 74
waist-to-hip ratio (WHR) 74
walking 69, 192–4, 209
Warm Cinnamon Apple Pudding 296–7
water intake 64, 177
white blood cells (leucocytes) 12–14, 17, 33, 135, 136, 154; *see also specific type*
Wild Rice Salad 261–2
wine, red 103
wound healing 21, 62, 123, 132, 148–9, 151, 161

xenobiotics 81

yeasts (in diet) 119–20, 124, 225
yoga 185–6, 199, 200–4
yoghurt 78, 101–2, 175, 225, **233**, **234**

Zesty Spinach Soup 253–4
zinc 54–5, 57, 151–2, 214, **234**